BREATHE

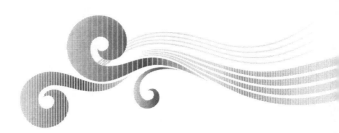

BREATHE

14 days to oxygenating,
recharging, and fueling
your body & brain

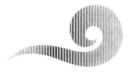

Dr. Belisa Vranich

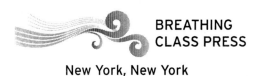
BREATHING
CLASS PRESS

New York, New York

BREATHE
By Belisa Vranich
Copyright © 2014 Belisa Vranich
thebreathingclass.com, Drbelisa@gmail.com, (646) 250-6390

Cover photograph: Caitlin Mitchell; Makeup: Janet Doman; Hair color: Naomi Strauss
Cover design: Wilbert Gutierrez; Retoucher: Gerald Echevarria
Anatomical still shot: Jeffrey Burns; Model: Mike Bell; Anatomical art: Hilary Mockewich
B-W images: Max Smith of Red Gremlin Design, and Shannon Orcutt
Research and editing: Jessica Cerretani
Publishing Coordinator: Simon Warwick-Smith of Warwick Associates
Legal: Anthony Gioffre and Robert Levine of Cuddy Feder, N.Y.
Website: Adam Furman of Saibot Technologies

Publisher's Cataloging-in-Publication
(Provided by Quality Books, Inc.)

Vranich, Belisa, 1966-
Breathe : 14 days to oxygenating, recharging, and
fueling your body & brain / by Dr. Belisa Vranich.
pages cm
LCCN 2013958265
ISBN 978-0-9913589-0-8
ISBN 978-0-9913589-1-5

1. Breathing exercises. 2. Meditation.
3. Relaxation. I. Title. II. Title: 14 days to
oxygenating, recharging, and fueling your body & brain.
III. Title: Fourteen days to oxygenating, recharging,
and fueling your body and brain.

RA782.V73 2014   613'.192
                        QBI14-600006

Simple as they may seem, before embarking on any exercise program, you should consult
with your medical doctor.

The exercises and practices in BREATHE are not intended to replace the services of your
physician or to provide an alternative to professional medical treatment. BREATHE offers
no diagnosis of or treatment for any specific medical problem that you may have. Where it
suggests the possible usefulness of certain practices in relation to certain illnesses or symptoms, it does so solely for educational purposes—either to explore the possible relationship
of natural breathing to health, or to expose the reader to alternative health and healing
approaches. The breathing practices outlined here are extremely gentle, and, if carried out
as described, should be beneficial to your overall physical and psychological health. If you
have any serious medical or psychological problems, such as heart disease, high blood pressure, cancer, mental illness, or recent abdominal or chest surgery, you should consult your
physician before undertaking these exercises.

"*Successful, long term weight loss needs you to address your stress/cortisol levels as cortisol causes your body to hold on to fat. Breathwork and meditation is the most successful way to do this, and Dr. Belisa teaches this in an easy, fast way. Lowering your stress and getting connected to your body is a critical part of a healthy lifestyle. Many of my clients have worked directly with Dr. Belisa and see immediate results in not just their waistline but in their overall happiness! Bravo, Belisa, for showing us how!*"

—LYN-GENET, author of New York Times bestseller *The Plan: Eliminate the Surprising "Healthy" Foods That Are Making You Fat – and Lose Weight Fast*

"*Most recently I utilized her expertise during a defensive tactics program conducted at the Manhattan DEA office. Dr. Belisa's reviews were outstanding. We trained approximately 30 Agents from the DEA and US Marshals Service. The feedback was fantastic.*"

—STEVE KARDIAN, former Chief Investigator, NYC Department of Investigation, New York

"*Women have fallen out of communication with their bodies and themselves. We have an epidemic of cancers and other life-threatening conditions that tug on the heartstrings of our civilization. If there's one educator leading the way to a clear and uncompromising understanding about women's health, it's Dr. Belisa.*"

—TERA WARNER, Director, Women's Summits for Health, Montreal, Canada

"Dr. Belisa's class helped alleviate my sciatica like no other treatment, so I was able to perform at Carnegie Hall once again! It is extraordinary."

—Ieva Siuksta, The Manhattan Symphonie Orchestra
Violinist, New York City

"I heard from so many consultants about how much they not only loved but needed your breathing class. You brought them to tears and made them laugh. It was such a unique class and I definitely want to make it staple for future events."

—PATTY BRISBEN, Pure Romance President and CEO, Inc 5000
and Fortune 500 Company, Cincinnati, Ohio

"Belisa is an incredibly open and gifted healer of others and her book is full of her amazing wisdom!"

—DAVID ELLIOT, Healer and author of Reluctant Healer and Healing

"The students raved about Dr. Belisa's class—it was well attended, and the students were thrilled to spend dedicated time with an expert who enabled them to concentrate on the root of much of their stress and technical problems."

—ANDREW HAUZE, Director,
Swarthmore College Orchestra and Wind Ensemble

"Dr. Belisa Vranich has developed a cutting-edge technique for reducing stress that translates well across cultures, and is proving to be effective with people who have been profoundly traumatized. Classic and groundbreaking, modern and ancient, it empowers as it heals."

—HAWTHORNE SMITH, PH.D., Bellevue/NYU Hospital

"A lightheaded, blissed-out state that, for some, borders on hallucinogenic. Even Xanax can't compare."

—KATIE BECKER, W Magazine

"I am in awe of the facility with which Dr. Belisa Vranich translates technical information about the body and breath into simple, fun, yet profound exercises to free life energy and restore health."

—JIM MORNINGSTAR, PH.D., Director, School of Integrative Psychology, Milwaukee, Wisconsin

"With her remarkable talent for making important health information poignant and practical, Dr. Belisa is a wealth of information like no other."

—LISA OZ, Radio and television personality, six-time *New York Times* Bestselling Author

"Groundbreaking in her summary of the importance of oxygen and breathing, Dr. Belisa tackles the deleterious effects of modern stress with boundless energy and enthusiasm."

—Martin Lindstrom, *New York Times* Bestselling Author and *Time Magazine's* "World's 100 Most Influential People" 2009

CONTENTS

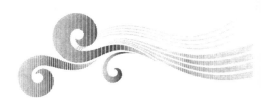

ACKNOWLEDGEMENTS

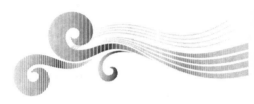

Concise though this book may be, don't let its simplicity and pithiness deceive you—years of energy, friendship, and work went into it and many friends and colleagues merit my heartfelt acknowledgements. To David Elliot, who started me on this journey, for his vision and love; to friends who enthusiastically supported *BREATHE* when, years ago, it was just a wisp of an idea: Sandra Guzman, Eva Huie, Tera Warner, Kristen Haines, Lyn-Genet, Joan Dallal, Amelia Hanibelsz, and Carmen Bedoya. Thank you, Alex Cohen, for your ruthless honesty and encouragement. Many, many thanks to my LA team: Karrie Wolfe and Heather Flores; my Philly team, Alma Qualli, of Osagame Martial Arts, Christine Levine, of Equal Fights Movement, and artistic genius Hilary Mockewich. My deepest gratitude for their time and feedback to Martin Lindstrom, Shirine Coburn, and Caitlin Mitchell, without whom I never would have persevered, and definitely wouldn't have finished; and to my NYC "siblings" Melissa Hobley and Sean Hyson for their enthusiasm

To Adam Furman, of Saibot, for his technical support and
friendship; Serena Lee for editing and ongoing emotional
support, Vernick Alvarez for his steadfast creative generosity, and Anthony Phillips for so many things that I lost
count. Heartfelt thanks to my yoga teachers past, present,
and future, but especially Monica Jaggi and Jules Febre. I
remain deeply grateful to Steve Kardian for his friendship
and generosity, and for his introduction to the wonderful
James Li and Mike DeBlaise. And wholehearted thanks for
friendship and support to Tricia Williams, Peder Regan, and
Jeffrey Burns of SciMedMedia, and to the tireless team at
Paul Wilmot Communications. Finally, to my colleagues
and friends at Willspace, thank you for embracing breathing
alongside squats and deadlifts.

PREFACE

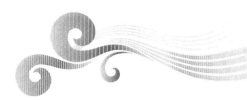

Too often you'll be told, "Just take a deep breath," so you take one dramatic, dysfunctional upper chest breath, then return to irregular shallow ones.

Too often you'll be told to slow down to breathe, or breathe to relax, or simply to belly breathe, with no more instruction than just that. If there is an explanation, it's too scanty to make sense anatomically, insufficient for it to gain traction in your mind as a habit you need to relearn.

Relearn—yes, thankfully learning to breathe efficiently is not a new habit you have to force into your life. You just have to remember (and not even consciously) how you used to breathe before you became an adult who sits for way too many hours a day, who has picked up bad habits because of back or shoulder or neck injuries, who is trying to suck in that gut and stand up straight, hence making your breathing the less efficient, anxiety-producing Vertical Breath that is so common now.

Nowadays, as compared to a few years ago, I rarely get

an utterly surprised look when I say I teach "breathing." More often than not, listeners leap into their own story of how they sense their own breath as being out of whack, and how they are looking for guidance. And then they are completely taken aback when I tell them that the opposite of "fight or flight" is "rest and digest." With the record-setting increase in incidences of sleep and digestive disorders today, it is not surprising that people don't know about "rest and digest." I believe that most of the gastrointestinal problems and sleep problems could be corrected by breathing better. Over and over my patients write to me the day following their initial session—they slept well!

Two names come to mind to me regularly when I teach. The father of modern medicine, Arthur Guyton, who says that the root of all physical and emotional suffering when broken down to the cellular level is low oxygen; and Dr. Andrew Weil, who advises that if you do only one thing for your health, have it be learning to breathe.

There are moments when breathing really does seem like a magic bullet. Throughout the past year I have never tired of hearing testimonials about how changing breathing to a more efficient, healthy-paced, and full body breath has changed someone's life: they don't have panic attacks anymore, they've quit smoking, their acid reflux is gone, their core is stronger, and they have more energy. Maybe the fatigue that you feel has to do with the lack of oxygen and the lack of balance of your breath—and if this is the case, your fast, shallow breathing needs a "makeover" right now.

The lesson in BREATHE, then, is to learn to breathe in a

way that is anatomically congruous and harmonious. It creates momentum so that you grasp "better breathing" quickly and whole-heartedly. "Dismantling"[1] the bad patterns and replacing them with those that make more "sense" to your body means breathing the way your body was designed to do—centered in the middle of your body—and taking better breaths.

BREATHE is a primer for all the breathing techniques you may learn in the future, be they yogic breath, breathing for optimal sports performance, breathing for anxiety relief, holotropic breathing or breathing in Pilates.

Take the time and effort to commit to planning 14 days to makeover your breathing. Whether you want to lower your cortisol (stress hormone), lose belly fat, or maximize the performance of your muscles and brain; or whether you are on a personal quest to be calmer and stress free, the first and most important step is: Breathe!

---

1. The concept of "dismantling" is from Donna Farhi's *The Breathing Book*.

HOW TO USE
THIS BOOK

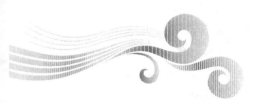

1. Get baseline measurements for yourself that are detailed
   in Chapter Two. You can use the form in the back of
   this book or note your baseline numbers and information on your own. As you try the exercises in the next
   few chapters, make notes about how many you can do
   or how difficult they feel. Your notes are important even
   if they are just descriptions (because essentially you can't
   see your lungs breathe and you can't see oxygen). If there
   are some exercises that you can't do or find awkward,
   just do your best and get an approximate baseline of your
   performance.

2. Make a workout for yourself exactly as you would with
   any exercise plan or weight-lifting routine at the gym.
   The baseline you have determined is the starting number.
   Make a commitment to focus on your lungs and breathing muscles every day for at least ten minutes. It doesn't

matter if you are doing this to address stress, to get ener-
gized, to get more oxygen to your muscles and organs so
you can sleep better, to heal faster, or to perform better.
What does matter is that you treat your workout like a
regimen for 14 days.

3. Determine your "max." This may mean that you can do
   40 Exhale Pulsations before you can't do anymore. Or
   it may mean that you do your Breathing Isometrics—a
   breathing count—2 minutes before you get jumbled up or
   distracted. That is OK. Just as with any exercise, you need
   to know what your starting point is and grow on that.

4. Don't get thrown by the idea that this is "just breathing." You are working out very important muscles in
   your body that have probably been idle. Feeling tired
   (maybe even perplexed because you haven't been running
   or lifting weights) is the result we are looking for. You
   are working internal muscles and there will be a moment
   where you hit your "max."

5. Treat the next 14 days like a health commitment that
   you cannot stray from. Make adjustments in your life
   to be able to dedicate at least ten minutes a day to your
   workout.

At some point over the next two weeks—it could be
on day two or it could be on day fourteen—your body will
"remember" what it has to do. You'll inhale from your
middle instead of your upper chest and it will feel surpris-
ingly natural. You'll notice your brain feels less foggy, you'll
know how to unwind at the end of the day, and whatever

hurts in your body will be alleviated or will have gone away all together. You may find in a few months that you need to reread parts of the book and take things up a notch, maybe do the harder exercises. Do a little refresher course and make the weights in *Roll Over Alligator* heavier or do a longer *Recovery Breath*.

You have much more control and power over how you feel than you realize. Taking control of your breathing will prove that to you.

INTRODUCTION

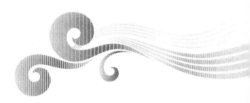

My interest in the mechanics of breathing was born a long time ago. As an adolescent I remember walking by my father on my way to the high school track as he did exhale pulsations ("Breath of Fire"). My father, unapologetically ahead of his time in many things, would meditate every day, the cat alongside him, in the living room. He routinely ran five miles a day in the early hours of the morning, but his enthusiasm for my running cross-country came from an unlikely place: his experience walking (and at times, running) from Yugoslavia to Italy in 1944, at age 12, with his mother and brother. He believed that being able to run was a gift that would keep me safe, keep me sane in times of stress, and keep me healthy. He ran every day late into life.

So I ran cross-country and track all through high school. Our coach even purchased a high-altitude tank that we would share and run with—making the average 5-mile runs even more excruciating. But we won state championships. Often. I continued running on my own in college. Then I took up boxing, practicing yoga, and lifting weights.

The bits of breathing we'd do in yoga fascinated me; however, I needed more extensive breathing exercises. Looking for classes, I went out west and studied in New Mexico and Los Angeles, finally finding different pockets of breathing methods. I looked up the history of breathing in medical documents, in sports. The internet was at that time peppered sparingly with information: an article on free diving, a video on Russian special operations training and breathing. I continued taking classes with breathworkers with all different levels of experience and sophistication. In training, my working would naturally combine my therapy background with my knowledge of breathing. Often loud, unexpected or intensely joyful or angry cathartic outbursts accompanied meditative states, but here there was less scientific knowledge for me to delve into, and more trust of the process.

My therapy and teaching background was always geared to understanding *why* and *how*. So when I taught, I focused on the *why* and the *how*; that is, the anatomy of lungs and the thoracic cavity, the psychology of anxiety and shallow breathing. People who would have never taken a breathing class in an alternative health or yoga setting discovered that breathing, which had seemed intangible and even fanciful, was very important—in fact, life-changing. Because of my love of martial arts, and perhaps the open-mindedness of the MMA community, the first dozen classes were at dojos and training centers, then with students at UCLA and Swarthmore, and also serendipitously, e.g., at a large corporate event for a company that sells sexual health products (now a yearly event).

My practice was transformed. From therapy with recommendation to do breathing/meditation, it became a breathing/meditation practice with hints of therapy. As a result, "mindfulness," once an elusive term for many, has become meaningful for people who have never been able to sit still, much less meditate. They can now meditate for ten, fifteen, twenty minutes at a stretch, and at times even more. They can hear themselves think, know how to center themselves, pick up on their intuition. They can do *Recovery Breath* in preparation for situations where they want to be focused, and they can decompress after a tough situation. They own their health. They find it incredibly empowering.

Given the intensity of the sessions and the unpredictable range of responses, I give thanks every day for a background of two decades in psychology. Breathwork has even greater implications and applications than I ever imagined. It heals. From the inside out.

So here you have it: Relearn to breathe. I can teach you. Dedicate 10 minutes a day for two weeks and notice a change in your energy level, your ability to relax, how your body feels and how your brain works.

Breathe!

ELEMENTS OF
BREATHING

*Oxygen is sustenance the way that food
can never be. Yes, you should eat leafy
greens, organic and local, take your
vitamins . . . but the best way to take
care of yourself is to deal with the most
important thing first: your breathing.
Everything else is secondary.*

DR. BELISA

You *know* your breathing could be better. Maybe it just gets "stuck" somewhere on the inhale, or you simply feel that you can never get enough air; or maybe you just sense in your gut that something is not quite right. You know how good a big, relaxing sigh and a deep, deep breath feel, and you wish you could hold that sensation longer. You may not know the first thing about respiration and pulmonary medicine past the plastic torso at your pediatrician's office, or the poster for the Heimlich maneuver at your favorite takeout that you stare at while waiting for your food, but the idea of "breathing better" resonates with you. You are curious.

What you *do* know, instinctively, is how it feels to be *out of breath*, either after running up a set of stairs or when you are panicked. You routinely experience that feeling of not being able to get a full breath, though you can't pinpoint when in your adult life it started, except that it's markedly different from how you used to breathe as a child, when you could hold your breath till you got to the very bottom of the pool, gulp in air and recover in seconds after sprinting, or yell at the top of your lungs seemingly endlessly. At that time in your life you were concerned with breathing only when you had a stuffy nose.

Recently you heard talk of breathing exercises, maybe as exercises for COPD or asthma, or as part of a yoga class. You may have brushed off the idea as trendy, like pole dancing or Tae Bo, but now there is a nagging feeling that yes, yes, actually that *is* something you'd like to try. Though you don't know how, you do know in your gut that improved breathing could help you feel better. Still, even the term "better" is vague. Perhaps it could energize you a little, rid you of the feeling of being tired all the time, or improve your memory. Maybe it could even help cut down the number of medications you are prescribed. And maybe, just maybe, it could help deal with the increasing stress in your life that—regardless of how many New Year's resolutions you devote to finding balance, taking time to relax, and being in the now—you can't get under control.

You shake your head and roll your eyes, thinking how pathetic you will sound telling your friends that you will call them back as soon as you are done with your breathing exercises. But then you think, what if this *is* the silver bullet? What if something this simple can make you healthier?

You are right. Your intuition is right. Your gut is right. Despite not being able to peer into your own chest, and knowing that the important stuff you inhale and exhale is totally invisible, you are absolutely, 100 percent right. It could lessen the pain or help you heal faster. Right. Help your digestive problems, be they acid reflux, irritable bowel, or constipation. Right again. Lower cortisol, making for easier weight loss. Lower blood pressure faster and more permanently than any medication on the market. You guessed it: right.

OXYGENATE FROM THE INSIDE OUT

Breathing: at first you might dismiss it as the stuff of pop songs by Faith Hill and Taylor Swift, but once you realize that oxygen is body fuel at a cellular level—it's how you nourish your brain and muscles—well, it starts making sense. A lot of sense.

And you do know this: you consider buying that face cream that professes to "oxygenate," you toy with the idea of taking supplements that assure "increased oxygenation" as well as drinking alkaline water that promises to lower your acidity. So now consider something you could do as quickly and more cheaply by adjusting your inhale and exhale, just a tad.

How well you breathe is the best indicator of how healthy you are, and how long you will live. "If I had to limit my advice on healthier living to *just one tip*," says Dr. Andrew Weil, "it would be simply to learn *how to breathe correctly*." The opposite is true as well, and even more extreme than you realize: "*All* chronic pain, suffering, and disease are caused by a lack of oxygen at the cell level . . . Proper breathing nourishes the cells of the body with oxygen, and optimizes the functioning of the body on all levels," states the eminent Dr. Arthur C. Guyton.[1] So why hasn't this been terribly evident to everyone? I'll give you three reasons:

1. *Can't see the forest for the trees.* Succinctly put, until you feel better, you don't realize how bad you were feeling before. Plus you can't really see the damage that is taking place. For example: your stomach doesn't feel good, and the upset is pretty obvious in your bowel movements (or lack thereof). With breathing and oxygen, the results are widespread throughout your entire body; however, lack of oxygen isn't something that cries out for immediate attention or needs a visible bandage or crutch. Face it, humans are very visual. The good news: the changes will be unquestionably evident after two weeks of doing the breathing exercises that I am going to outline.

2. *Not going to the source.* Medical care usually makes us feel better right away with a pill, a shot or sur-

---

1. Dr. Guyton's book, *Textbook of Medical Physiology*, is a household name in medical schools.

gery—but it doesn't go to the source of the problem. As a society, we're neither accustomed nor taught to search for the root of the problem and solve it from there. Take blood pressure, for example: medication is highly effective whereas breathing exercises are just as effective for lowering it without side effects by going to the source (in this case, over-arousal of the sympathetic nervous system).

3. *The fight or flight response got stuck.* The change from the healthy breathing of a child to the dysfunctional breathing of an adult could creep in over the years. A bad fright in adolescence, for example, could change one's breathing from full to shallow. And this shallow breathing, reinforced by a hunched posture that is the result of years of sitting at a desk or driving, could become ingrained. A stressful event, followed by a back injury as a young adult could lead to dysfunctional breathing, which becomes a habit after a few years; then stress and a culture of "gut-sucking" leads to sipping air haltingly, not exhaling completely, never getting as much oxygen as needed in order to think clearly and sleep well.

WE HAVE EVOLVED, BUT OUR BREATHING HAS "DE-VOLVED"

Lung capacity and inhale/exhale strength are two of the few human capacities that have actually 'devolved' over time. Not to mean that we are turning back into fish, but rather that our breathing has become incrementally dysfunctional.

While our brains have gotten bigger and we have the potential to live to 120—even to break records in speed and capacity in sports every year—most of us "under-breathe" or breathe in a dysfunctional way.

In part this comes from what I call "Illnesses of Too Fast": we walk faster than we did 10 years ago, eat faster, communicate faster, and actually age faster when exposed to oxidative stress for too long a time. Even acid reflux can come from swallowing too fast, then jumping to the next task. We are under constant pressure to go to sleep quickly and to wake up quickly. And, consequently, what happens? Our breathing is constantly in "fast mode," shallow and quick, which in turn has terrible health repercussions.

You get it; it makes sense. Many illnesses are caused or made worse by lack or imbalance of oxygen. Your system may be too acidic or inflammatory, perhaps you're carrying stubborn pounds that won't come off because of high cortisol, or you're suffering from memory problems owing to an oxygen-starved brain. And yes, your energy level is low because you don't fuel your cells with the one thing they need: oxygen. With the one thing that they need to make all that expensive organic food and supplements digestible: oxygen. Every time you breathe, you nourish your body and brain. So why don't you start to feed it better? You can deal with it now.

THE ULTIMATE ANSWER TO STRESS

This book is the ultimate answer to stress. It will give you guidelines to turn your life around in 14 days. It will teach you *to control stress—not let it control you.* How?

- By activating your underutilized diaphragm muscle.
- By deactivating dysfunctional breathing patterns.
- By realigning your breathing to work with your body, not against it.
- By working your breathing muscles just as you would in physical therapy.
- By determining your baseline numbers for stress, blood pressure, pain, sleeplessness, and fatigue.

So revitalize, rejuvenate and feel better than ever before!

CAN THIS BOOK REPLACE A BREATHING CLASS?

And what is a "breathing class anyway"? It is an exercise class (you'll sweat!) for your lungs; it's a meditation-for-people-who-can't meditate class. It deals with anatomy and psychology, it can lower your blood pressure, address your constipation, get you oxygenated faster—better than any medications. (Even for athletes, it is a secret weapon. They don't need more cardio for their endurance; they need this book.) Breathing exercises can energize you better than a Red Bull, put you to sleep better than an Ambien. They are the number one antidote for stress: lowering your blood pressure, cortisol, and neutralizing your acidity in minutes. If you do one thing for your health this year, let it be retraining yourself to breathe in a way that nourishes your body *at a cellular level.*

HOW BAD IS MY BREATHING?

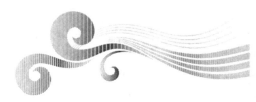

> *How one breathes is an indicator of longevity and quality of life. The health of your body is reflected in the way you breathe. Change the way you breathe and there will automatically be positive changes in your longevity and quality of life.*[1]
>
> DR. BELISA

WORRIED? YOU SHOULD BE

Poor breathing puts you at higher risk for a slew of diseases and problems. Here are 4 biggies.

---

1. The renowned Framingham study presented persuasive evidence that the most significant factor in health and longevity is how well one breathes. The complete study can be accessed at the National Institute of Health's Database: http://www.ncbi.nlm.nih.gov/PubMed/.

- *Back pain.* Mild oxygen deprivation can cause or contribute to back pain, according to Dr. John E. Sarno, an expert on back problems and author of New York Times bestseller *Healing Back Pain.*
- *High blood pressure.* Sub-optimal breathing may contribute to hypertension. In a nutshell, faster breathing results in acidic blood and decreased ability to pump out more sodium, which raises blood pressure. The opposite is also true: people with HBP who were made to breathe slower several minutes a day saw their blood pressure drop.[2]
- *Digestive woes.* Optimally, your breathing muscles should stimulate "peristalsis," the wavelike motion of the intestines that promotes digestion and elimination. Without this internal abdominal massage, you're likely to find yourself coping with constipation, bloating, gas, heartburn, and irritable bowel syndrome.
- *Cognitive and emotional problems.* Insufficient oxygen makes concentration difficult, causes problems with memory, and results in low energy levels. Both depression and anxiety are worsened by shallow, erratic breathing.

IT'S NOT JUST ABOUT CARDIO

You find yourself gasping for air after climbing a few flights of stairs and automatically think, "I really need to do more

---

2. For more specifics, go to:

http://www.ncbi.nlm.nih.gov pubmed/10205248/;

and http://www.ncbi.nlm.nih.gov/pmc/articles/PMC2288755/.

cardio." It's true that cardio—or aerobic exercise—is crucial in keeping you healthy. It is a type of activity that can strengthen your heart muscle by improving its ability to pump blood (and oxygen) throughout the body. Cardio can have a bevy of benefits, *but your heart can only move as much oxygen as you bring into your body.* Here's the crux of the problem: cardio exercise gives your heart a great workout, but it does nothing to beef up the power of your lungs, improve the flexibility of your thoracic cavity (the bones, tendons, cartilage, and muscles that make up the chest wall), or strengthen your inspiratory and expiratory muscles, and the thoracic diaphragm. In other words, you can have the heart and cardiovascular system of an elite athlete but the lungs and breathing muscles of a total couch potato. Just because you train until you are sweating up a storm and heaving for breath doesn't mean you are actually working out the specific components that make for better breathing.

> If you have cardiovascular disease, one of the best things you can do is learn how to breathe better, in order to give your heart a break. A lower resting heart rate, which you can learn to induce yourself with your breath, means your whole system can rest and heal.

A GREAT PAIR OF LUNGS

You might not think much about your lungs until you're short of breath or have a condition like asthma that affects their function. But these seemingly ordinary organs have the power to determine whether or not you are supplying your brain and body with the sustenance they need. The very purpose of the lungs is to draw in oxygen and remove carbon dioxide from your body. And keeping this balance is exactly what your body needs to be alert, productive, and happy.

OXYGEN IS CELL FOOD

Stop and consider how much money you spend on vitamins, green juices, and the newest electrolyte-infused alkaline neutral water. However, what it comes down to when all is said and done, is that your body's main source of energy is *oxygen*. Period. As oxygen circulates throughout your system, it is released into the cells in your tissues and organs, where it can interact with certain enzymes, creating fuel for your body. Oxygen, then, is vital for the respiration and growth of healthy cells—the very cells that allow you to think, the cells that break down your food, the cells that produce balancing hormones and neurotransmitters. Without those hard-working cells, you will find yourself reaching for supplements, energy drinks, and medications to help you feel better. And the real solution is right under your nose.

Imagine needing only two breaths instead of ten in order to catch your breath. *And* being able to push yourself more during your workouts *and* recover more quickly afterward. *And* your energy levels will naturally be higher. *And* you'll be able to think more clearly and recall more precisely. That's the promise of optimal oxygen intake—and it's something you can achieve by working out your breathing muscles.

PUMPING OXYGEN

Sure enough, it seems that everyone has a solution for increasing oxygen in the body, from altitude training, oxygen tents, eating a diet that's low in salt and rich in alkaline foods (which supposedly changes the pH of your body to one that encourages oxygenation), to drinking ionized water or huffing canned oxygen. They also propose popping supplements said to improve the ability of red blood cells to bind with oxygen (such as folate, chlorophyll, algae, and vitamins A, B6, B12, and C), sleeping in oxygen-deprived tanks, or even wearing mouth devices that restrict airflow and hence work your lungs. But before you rush out to GMC or start filling your virtual Amazon.com cart with pricey gadgets and gizmos, consider this: You can most certainly add oxygen to your blood, but the boost it gives you—if it does—is fleeting. Why not improve the way you breathe, all the time?

A BETTER WAY TO BOOST OXYGEN

So forget about oxygen-boosting products. There is a better way—and I will teach it to you. Moreover, its effects are permanent (and free).

If you have ever seen cadaver studies of lungs, you must have been amazed at how far these organs can stretch (and if you haven't, head on over to YouTube right now for some mind-blowing images). The fact is, people use very little of all that lung space. That's because they are lazy breathers—taking short, shallow breaths from the chest, filling only the very top portion of the lungs with air. Then they do not exhale fully (with most breaths, 30 percent of stale air stays in the body). A rigid, inflexible thoracic cavity and ribcage, plus poor posture, also contribute to sluggish breathing.

The good news? While your parents (or, more accurately, their genes) are responsible for the size of your lungs, that doesn't mean you can't pump up their power. Let's take the first step right now.

DETERMINING YOUR BASELINE

Improving your breathing is just the same as working any other part of your body. You have a baseline and you work up from there. Just because you can't see your lungs working or can't see the air that comes in and goes out of them doesn't mean you can't measure your progress. In fact, it's critical that you do. I will help you determine your baseline.[3]

1. Vital lung capacity: wrap a measuring tape an inch beneath your sternum. Your sternum (breastbone) is a long flat bony plate shaped like a capital "T" that connects to the rib bones via cartilage. You may feel a "notch" where your ribs curl up and meet in the very middle of your chest. Exhale and measure the circumference of your body. Then inhale and measure. Do not change the way you breathe in order to make this

---

3. See "Establish Your Baseline" form at the end of this book. *After two weeks of doing the breathing exercises, retake these measurements. Detailed information on what each one of these means can be found online at www.thebreathingclass.com*

number change; simply breathe the way you do nor-
mally.[4]

2. Breathhold: this measure can only be taken only once,
   at the very beginning. It is used to establish a baseline,
   and then to check your progress in two weeks. Mul-
   tiple measurements will confuse the results because it's
   not a reliable method for tracking change over time.
   Once you start retesting, it becomes a test in itself to
   see how long you can hold your breath, how much
   discomfort in the breathhold you can tolerate. Not
   our goal. Hold your breath now for as long as you
   can and note that number. This number is important
   because it gives you a general sense of how much oxygen there is in your body (or how well balanced your
   oxygen and carbon dioxide are).[5]

3. Number of breaths per minute: have someone watch
   you breathe when you are focusing on something else.
   Have them note how many breaths you take in 15
   seconds, then multiply by 4. They should also note the
   quality of your breathing if possible. How long is the
   inhale as compared to the exhale? Note where you feel
   resistance, as if you are "sticking" on the inhale.

---

4. For a visual on measuring lung capacity, check out chiropractor Dr. Paula
Moore's video on http://www.youtube.com/watch?v=8G-HVCOYTGw.

5. Please note: If you have orthostatic hypotension, hypertension, heart
issues, or COPD, holding your breath (no oxygen and more co2) may not
be safe depending on how severe your case is. Skip this measure until you
are cleared by your doctor or have resolved the issue.

4. Resting heart rate: take these measurements and note them on day one. Then again on day 14. To find your resting heart rate, press the index and middle fingers over the underside of the opposite wrist, just below the thumb. To find the pulse on the side of the neck, place your index and middle finger in the hollow between the windpipe and the large muscle in the neck. Count the beats for one minute, or count for 30 seconds and multiply by two, or count for 15 seconds and multiply by four. To ensure an accurate reading, sit quietly for several minutes before taking your pulse.

5. Stress: on a scale of 1-10, with *ten* being the most stress, how stressed are you now? Over the past week, what was your average stress level? Over the last month? Do not judge your stress by the events that caused them. Stress can be caused by worries about an impending problem; they are not necessarily the result of a direct trauma. This is a subjective number that has to do only with you. Over the next 14 days, rate your stress.

6. Pain: if you are experiencing pain of any type, from fibromyalgia to back pain, rate your pain as well. 1 is no pain, 5 is average (tolerable), 10 is acute. As with #5 above, do not judge whether your pain "deserves" a certain number or should be higher or lower; simply rate it by how it feels to you—regardless of whether you have a high or low pain threshold.

7. Energy level: while your energy level may fluctuate throughout the day, rate your level on an average

as compared to prior days. Start by noting how you remember it being last week and the previous month. Give each day a number for the next 14 days.

8. Sleep: if you under-breathe, it's quite possible that your sleep is affected. Do you have difficulty going to sleep or staying asleep? If you have trouble "turning off the chatter"—the running commentary in your head that keeps you up at night—rate how severe your sleep problems are.[6] If you take medication to help get you to sleep, rate this problem a 10.

9. Mood: rate your mood last week, and last month. If you have had specific changes in your mood (depression or anxiety), note when they started and record any fluctuations in severity. Then, every day over the next two weeks measure your mood. Remember that a higher number means a severe upset in your depression or anxiety. A 1 or 2 would be a very good day, with little or no symptoms of depression or anxiety, while a 10 would be one where you would consider seeking ER care.

10. Endurance: pick a measure for your endurance, whether it be when going up a set of stairs you take every day or a five-mile run you do several times a month. Factor out the quality of your day or your energy level, and strive to get a clear sense of how

---

6. Anxiety will cause you to have low GABA, which means your mind will continue to race at night. High cortisol and low progesterone are also culprits.

your endurance changes as you do these exercises over the next few days. The number in this case is very subjective and should reflect how you assess your conditioning (ability to catch your breath) that day.

11. Cravings: If weight loss is an issue with you, give your feelings of hunger or cravings a number. Again 1 is none, while 10 is intolerable. Note your history with feelings of hunger and cravings over the last month and the last year in general. Note the time of the craving and type of food as well.

12. Are you a Vertical or Horizontal Breather?

13. Describe and rate your neck and shoulder stiffness/discomfort.

14. Describe and rate your sense of mental clarity and memory.

15. Describe and rate any problems with your digestion including not emptying your bowels once a day, acid reflux/heartburn, irritable bowel syndrome.[7] Include any pelvic floor problem; e.g., light leakage, incontinence or urgency if it's applicable.

---

7. According to Dr. Robert Zembroski of the Darien Center for Functional Medicine, "If you have difficulty with bowel movements and a lack of motility, consider investigating your hormones. Thyroid weakness is a common cause of constipation. If you are tired of chewing Tums or taking an antacid, first and foremost change your diet. Dairy and grain are common food irritants that can cause a multitude of miserable symptoms including reflux and heartburn, bloating, and loose stools."

EVERYONE
UNDER-BREATHES

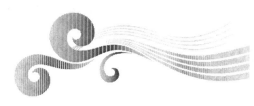

*It speaks volumes that we all know what
'fight or flight' is but we don't know what
the opposite is. Do you? It's 'rest and
digest.' In order to live a healthy life, you
need both. Right now most of us stay in
'fight or flight,' as if we didn't have an
alternative. No wonder we can't sleep and
we have so many digestive problems: not
enough 'rest and digest'!*

DR. BELISA

Owing to any number of influences, very few people breathe
to their full potential. I see this time and time again in the
breathing classes I teach. A new client comes to me and
reports that she is eating clean, drinking more water, popping supplements, seeing the chiropractor and using a heat-

ing pad to keep old injuries at bay and icing new ones. She is doing everything right.

Then I ask her one simple question: *How is your breathing?* And she points to her nose and tells me about her allergies.

I'm sure you can relate. But did you know that just about anything and everything—from your age, your health history, to your texting addiction—can have a powerful impact on your capacity to breathe optimally? In this chapter, I'd like you to assess how you actually breathe now and to consider the possibility that you're not breathing as well as you should—in everyday life, on the treadmill, at the computer.

SELF-EXAM: LET'S LOOK AT YOU

Still think you're breathing as well as you could? Well, think again—and answer the ten questions I ask everyone:

1. Do you sit in front of a computer or in a car or truck for work?
2. Do you wear Spanx, support pantyhose, or a bulletproof vest?
3. As a child, did you live with any type of fear, anxiety, or worry over a period of time, even if you think you weren't traumatized by it?
4. Do you text throughout the day?
5. Do you carry a bag, knapsack, purse? How much does it weigh?
6. Have you ever had pneumonia or recurring bouts of bronchitis?
7. Have you ever smoked or lived with a smoker?

8. Have you ever lived or spent time in a city with high levels of smog or pollution, or lived someplace with noxious smells?

9. Do you have a deviated septum or do you snore?

10. Do you have or have you ever had neck, shoulder, or back injuries?

Oh, and are you over age 29?[1]

How many questions did you say *yes* to? Even just one of these can lead to under-breathing, either by impairing lung function or laying the foundation for one or more of the abnormal breathing patterns to be discussed in this chapter. So if you are breathing poorly—and you probably are—you could be doing so for any number of reasons, apart from those mentioned in the quiz. These include:

• Chronic stress, anxiety, or a history of panic attacks or other anxiety disorders. Before you dismiss these as "not me," think about whether you have ever stayed awake worrying about money, your health, the stress of a divorce or breakup, the care of your kids, or being the caretaker of elderly parents. If any one of these sounds familiar, chances are, you're stressed out.

• Technology and poor posture. Think your posture is fine? How many times a day do you bend your head to text, to update your Facebook status, or play a game on your phone? How many hours are you hunched

---

1. Yup, even your age affects your breathing. It might be said that things improve with time, but lung function isn't one of them—it naturally heads downhill after age 29.

over a laptop or desk? These positions put your head and shoulders into a position that impairs breathing up to 30 percent.[2]

- Long periods of time spent sitting down, whether while driving, working, or watching TV. The latest studies of how many hours people sit a day report an average of 13 hours.[3]
- Anything around your waist: a tool belt, or just your average waistband that holds your pants or skirt around your middle.
- Lung or nose issues. Deviated septum or broken nose, snoring, allergies or sinus problems, asthma, emphysema, and other respiratory diseases.
- Your body. Beer belly, extra abdominal weight. Neck, shoulder, or back injuries, *past* and present.

ABNORMAL BREATHING PATTERNS

Pause a moment and pay attention to your breath without trying to influence it. Now think about how you breathe in more challenging situations; e.g., during a workout or a jog. Are you using the right muscles to breathe? Are you filling just part of your lungs with oxygen-rich air? Chances

---

2. According to chiropractors and other experts, dysfunctional breathing is intimately involved in back, neck, and shoulder pain. Likewise, poor posture (often the result of pain) can worsen breathing patterns. It's a vicious cycle that you need to break in order to achieve optimal breathing.

3. Check out: http://www.prnewswire.com/news-releases/new-survey-to-sit-or-stand-almost-70-of-full-time-american-workers-hate-sitting-but-they-do-it-all-day-every-day-215804771.html.

are you're stuck in one of the following abnormal breathing patterns. In the last chapter you noted if you were a "Horizontal" or "Vertical" Breather (breathing up and down or widening when you inhale and exhale). Now look more specifically: which of the following types sound familiar?

- *Clavicular breathing.* This common form of inefficient breathing fills only the top part of your lungs, using the muscles in your neck and shoulders to inhale. Have someone watch you while you breathe: do your shoulders move up slightly or do you feel your collarbones rise as you inhale? If you are a "clavicular" breather, you actually end up using more energy breathing this way, often tiring faster even though you are taking in big gulps of air.
- *Paradoxical breathing.* Also known as "reverse breathing," this pattern uses your muscles in a contradictory manner; this is to say, you draw your belly in during an inhale and relax it out during an exhale—the polar opposite of what you should be doing. Paradoxical breathers take in significantly less air than anyone else, actually going against what their body wants to do, anatomically, with each inhale and exhale. Theory says that it comes from anxiety in childhood—try gasping in fear and see how you mimic that breathing.
- *Periodic breathing.* Another stress-fueled pattern, periodic breathing combines breath-holding and heavy sighing. This abnormal cycle is your body's over-eager attempt to raise and lower levels of carbon dioxide in the bloodstream.

- *Breath-holding.* This abnormal pattern (also called hypoxic breathing) is alarmingly common. My clients have reported being surprised as they find themselves holding their breath for several seconds throughout the day for no apparent reason. This pattern throws whatever balance you may have out of whack, as your body continuously tries to compensate for the moments in which you are not letting carbon dioxide out or oxygen in.

- *Over-breathing.* Chronic ventilation at low levels results in an imbalance of carbon dioxide and oxygen. Although you're breathing more quickly, you are out of balance. There are two breakdowns here: your exhale is strong and your inhale is constricted, or the opposite, your inhale is long and your exhale is short.

Now that you know the many different types of abnormal breathing patterns and the factors that can influence how you breathe, you can see why virtually no one these days breathes optimally without proper training.

Watch a baby breathe, and you'll witness the perfect breath: gentle, relaxed, rhythmic, with the belly expanding horizontally, and little movement in the collarbone or shoulders. Yet very few people sustain that perfection into adulthood. Bad posture, injury, and just plain laziness lead them to the mediocre-at-best breathing they practice now. In essence, they're breathing the way our ancestors did when they were faced with fear, anxiety, or other *temporary* situations. Unfortunately, we've transformed these short-term solutions into long-term abnormal breathing patterns.

I know what you're thinking: *Okay, so my breathing is terrible! Now what?* Well, now I'm going to show you why abnormal breathing patterns don't have to be "normal" for you—and how you can make every breath count.

WARM UP,
EXHALE FIRST

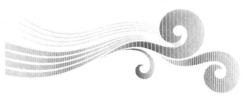

*Just the attention that you are paying to
your breathing, just the awareness you are
bringing to it a few times a day, sporadically,
means you have started to change—to get
better. You are taking in more air than
yesterday, even if all you are doing is
noticing your breath from time to time.*

DR. BELISA

When you pack your knapsack or suitcase most efficiently,
you use up every little crack and cranny, shifting things
around to maximize space. This is what you are going to do
with your lungs, which may even result in your growing new
lung tissue! The truth is, even if you have Aquaman-sized
lungs, it matters little if the muscles that form your thoracic
cavity—also known as your inspiratory and expiratory
muscles—aren't strong and flexible. These muscles, which

include the ones between each and every rib, on the inside *and* on the outside, help you inhale and exhale to your full potential. This chapter and the next will help you utilize the maximum capacity of your lungs and ensure that the encasement of your lungs is as flexible as possible in order to help, not hinder, your breathing. For a visual, see pages 52–55. The exercises in this chapter will set you on your path to better health and performance by helping you rethink your own respiration. And it's as simple as transforming the most basic components of a breath: your inhalations and exhalations.

EXHALE MAXIMIZATIONS

First, let's work on your exhale. This may seem counterintuitive: When you think about breathing, it's probable that your mind automatically goes to your inhale because it's what takes in much-needed oxygen. In fact, most people barely exhale at all, let alone fully; yet mediocre exhalations are a major contributor to poor breathing.

You see, between each breath, a whopping 20 to 30 percent of air stays in your lungs, just settling there and getting stale (and if you are a really lazy exhaler, it may be even more). The result is that these organs can't expand to their full capacity with fresh air on your next inhalation. In other words, your starting inhalations *have* to be less than optimal.[1]

---

1. During inspiration, an estimated 500 mL of "fresh" atmospheric air enters your body, but only the first 350 mL actually reaches the alveoli in your lungs. In fact, the remaining 150 mL stays in your nose, pharynx, larynx, trachea, and other airways without alveoli—basically, dead space.

With the following exercises, I'm going to show you how to squeeze out as much of that stale air as possible on your exhales, so there will be plenty of room in your lungs for new, oxygen-rich air. Recognize that your inhale and your exhale are not just the same mechanism in reverse order. Your inhale is governed primarily by the flattening out of your diaphragm, which pulls in air. Your exhale is usually even more passive: You just stop inhaling and "let the air out" as you would let it out of a balloon. So let's work on making that better.

1. Start by taking a normal breath, that is, exactly like the one you took just before you started reading this. Don't make this one "better" because now you are paying attention! Simply notice how you take in air until you meet some resistance in the inhale and stop; then your exhale is really just a letting go. Notice how passive this is. Imagine how much air you are taking in. The average is 12 ounces, or a cup and a half. If you had to measure the amount of air you inhale and exhale, it might be even less, maybe it would be half a cup, or even a few tablespoons—especially if you are sitting and concentrating in such a way that you completely disconnect from your body, like while at a computer or driving.

2. On your next exhale, put some attention into the emp-

Make no mistake: your alveoli do fill with 500 mL of air, but only two-thirds of it is fresh because 150 mL is already sitting in there, getting stale. No wonder most people aren't getting all the oxygen they need.

tying of air. Tighten your abs in an attempt to really squeeze out all the stale air. Does working your abs at the same time count as multitasking? Absolutely. It's not the ab muscles that give you a six-pack; in effect, there are more important ones deeper inside that have to do with core and pelvic stability.

3. Take it up a notch: On your next exhale, squeeze the last bit of air out with your core and ab muscles. And don't stop at a neutral (flat) stomach. Actually go one step further (to a bowl shape); you might even push your fingers into your stomach and around your ribcage to become completely aware of the mechanics of this. (Prone on your back or leaning over works best when you are starting out because of gravity.) Finally, scrunch up your face and pretend you are blowing out of a small straw. Don't worry if you cough a little. Then try "Lion's Breath," which means sticking your tongue out on the exhale. Notice how much air was left over from your normal lazy exhale compared to your more attentive one. Think of all the wasted space that you could fill with clean air.

4. Take 5 normal breaths, focusing intently on the exhale. On the next 5 breaths, concentrate on taking a really big inhale. Notice how your inhale is automatically a bigger, more efficient breath because you have emptied out beforehand. Compare this breath to the one before in terms of efficacy. Remember that stale air stays in your lungs unless you consciously exhale it. Just keep training yourself to blow out every last little bit.

Do this: Barely exhale, then go to your inhale. Continue another 5 or 6 breaths like this, having your exhale be only a fraction of your inhale. Notice how it is possible to continue breathing in this way. Become aware that given injuries, posture, and bad habits, it would be easy to fall into the trap of always breathing this way (on a much more subtle level, of course). Now think about the math, think about breathing this way for months, for years. Despite feeling as if you are taking a deep breath, the actual exchange of oxygen and carbon dioxide is completely out of balance, and your inhale is very shallow.

Listen up: 80 percent of your lung capacity is in your sides and back! The next stage in maximizing your inhalations is to consider how well your breath reflects the flexibility of your thoracic cavity. If you sit at a desk at work or spend several hours a day in a car, then it's probably pretty darn rigid. The size of your lungs doesn't even matter: If the receptacle that holds them is stiff and unyielding, it won't let you get much air in. Making the muscles in your sides and back, between your ribs—your intercostal muscles—more flexible means they will expand more, allowing you to take a bigger breath. Now you are ready to move on to a sitting, and then a standing Intercostal Stretch, followed by an Intercostal Crunch.

1. Sitting up straight, drape one arm over your head so that the bicep is covering your ear. Visualizing the little muscles in between each rib right under your armpit, stretch over to the opposite direction, keeping your elbow straight up. Do not hold your

breath. Inhale during
the stretch and exhale
when you relax a bit
or come up. If this
stretch is easy for you,
add some awareness
to the opposite side,

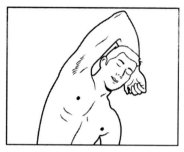

doing an "Intercostal Crunch." Then reverse sides.

2. This stretch can be done standing next to the wall as well, with one palm on the wall. The arm closest to the wall should stretch down towards your knee as you feel the stretch in your ribcage. If you have a high tolerance for pain, do not do these exercises to the top of your pain threshold because you don't want to injure your intercostal muscles.

3. While seated, pretend to hold a large medicine ball in front of you. Stretch your arms over the ball on the inhale and relax on the exhale. Bring attention to your back. The front of your body should hollow out, making space for the imaginary ball. Imagine the

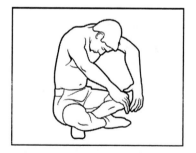

intercostal muscles stretching in your back. Keep in mind that most of your lung capacity is in your sides and back. Try to "puff up your back" on the inhale. Remind yourself that your lungs stretch down much farther in the back than in the front.

To get your thoracic cavity to be more flexible, do the side-to-side stretches on the floor. Remember that the "Intercostal Crunches" are the side stretches where you bring awareness to the side that is collapsing, in addition to the one that is stretching. There will be subtleties in stretching at the joint (which I definitely don't want you to do), versus stretching the muscles between your ribs. See if you can focus below your armpit, more along your sides.[2] The "crunch" on the opposite side is just as important.

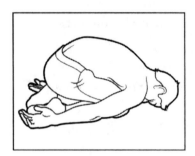

Do the *Child's Pose* to bring awareness to your back. Remember, your chin should almost fit between your knees; keep arms back with shoulders "melting" down as you relax with each breath.[3]

After having done these warm-up exercises and stretches, your vital lung capacity will already have improved. (This can be measured by breathing into a balloon or by measuring around your middle with a fabric measuring tape pre- and post-exercise.) Bring aware-

---

2. For increasing chest wall expansion, see: http://psychcentral.com/news/archives/2006-04/aps-syt033006.html.

3. If you have difficulty pointing your toes back or dropping your head low enough to get to the floor, or have trouble with your lower back, try a supported *Child's Pose*: put a rounded pillow or bolster horizontally from your tummy to head, or between your calves and butt to lessen the pressure if you are still too stiff or need the extra support.

ness to how far you can get on your first attempt. After having done the stretches, repeat the Inhale and Exhale Maximizations, and notice a change in the depth of both.

REFINING YOUR MOVES

1. When you are on your back, hold a 6-, 8- or 10-pound weight on your stomach (or, if you feel as if you can handle it, use a small kettlebell) and see how far you can let it fall into your stomach as you exhale. You might want to pick a heavier weight because this is not about raising it, but about seeing how close you can get your belly to your spine. Be careful not to bounce the weight.

2. Sit up, seeing how close you can come to keeping that "bowl" shape while sitting. After you have worked on these expiration muscles for a while, you will be able to maintain that concave bowl shape in your middle. When you are doing Exhale Maximizations, try to mimic the amount of "inward" curve you can get with the weight.

3. Does exhaling and contracting your stomach not seem natural? In order to relearn this (because you used to breathe this way as a baby), cough and see which way your belly goes. I bet you it contracts and pulls in, right? Keep this in mind when as you retrain your body. More on this in the next chapter.

ACTIVATE AND RELEARN

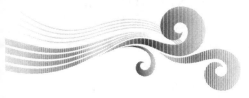

This isn't really a brand new skill you have to learn; you used to do it right. It's just about remembering. So simply put, while you may still breathe in a dysfunctional, that is, in a wrong way, don't worry; you don't have to put breathing on that endless list of to-do's that require breaking down a habit or painfully reminding yourself daily about a new one. It is simply about moving your breath down to the lower part of your body, where it used to be. Where it should be.

DR. BELISA

You've seen those ads for antihistamines or air fresheners in which a model spreads her arms wide, twirling in a circle, and expanding her chest, takes a deep, deep breath and sighs

blissfully. In another scenario a coach will tell an athlete
to breathe deeply. In most cases the shoulders either move
back or up. Unfortunately, this upper chest or clavicular
breathing is not efficient; it uses only the smaller top part
of your lungs, and that means that your diaphragm, which
should be your main breathing muscle, is completely still.
Bad, bad breathing.

Now, put one hand on your belly and one hand by
your collarbones. Open your mouth, close your eyes and
take a couple of breaths. *Notice which hand moves.* Is your
top hand moving up and down slightly, or is your bottom
hand moving forward and back? Maybe you aren't sure of
the direction, but you do know that one hand is moving
more than the other. Or perhaps they are both moving, just
a little bit. Ask someone to watch you breathe as you focus
on something else. Are they seeing one hand move more
than the other? Or is it a combination of belly *and* upper
chest movement?

Got neck or shoulder pain? When you are breathing through the top of
your body, you are using neck and shoulder muscles that are not meant
to be primary breathing muscles. Hence no matter how many massages
you have, how many therapeutic pillows or ergonomic chairs you buy,
you'll continue to have neck and shoulder discomfort until you change
your breathing back to the right way. The good news: Once you change
your breathing, your neck and shoulder stiffness will get better, and
stay better.

MEET YOUR DIAPHRAGM

The most important and underappreciated muscle in your body is the diaphragm.[1] If you've heard about the diaphragm, you probably have a vague idea that singers use it when reaching for a high C, but that's about it. In fact, this large, pizza-sized muscle plays an integral role in respiration. When you're not breathing with your diaphragm—and consequently not using the rest of your breathing muscles to their full potential—you're breathing just enough to survive, *but not enough to thrive.* For a visual, see pages 50–51.

In simplest terms, when you breathe properly—from the belly—your diaphragm flattens and spreads, and your bottom ribs and abdomen push out. Often the tired-can't-breathe sensation you may have experienced is due to those very muscles fatiguing; however, since the sensation is not as specific as the burn in your calves or biceps when you are working out at the gym, you don't recognize it as signaling underdeveloped breathing muscles.

Don't worry if you feel silly pushing your belly in and out. Once you get more advanced, your middle will simply widen. It will also contract more than before on the exhale. The result, when you do want to suck in your gut for a picture or do anything that involves your core muscles, you'll be able to do it better, for longer!

However, the diaphragm is just one major player in the game plan of breathing correctly. It's smack in the center of your body, surrounded and supported by the erector spinae, transverse abdominis, and

---

1. For an excellent article on the diaphragm, see:
http://www.dynamicchiropractic.com/mpacms/dc/article.php?id=55951

pelvic floor muscles. Your intercostals are also integral to respiration, while your outer core—the rectus abdominus, quadratus lumborum, and oblique muscles—help control your posture and movement. Never forget: strong breathing is a lot more than just the size of your lungs or how much cardio (heart exercise) you do!

When your diaphragm and other specific breathing muscles aren't as strong as they should be, your breathing suffers. In fact, right now these muscles are probably downright weak. Not to worry, though: I'm going to challenge you to work your diaphragm and core as you never have before—and all without lifting a dumbbell or doing a crunch.

RELEARN HOW TO BREATHE - SWITCHING BACK TO LOWER BODY BREATHING (LBB)

Babies have the most efficient, most centering breaths. So how does one go from a perfectly breathing infant to a poorly breathing adult? Well, as people get older, they sit for hours at desks, on sofas, on trains, and in cars—and these sustained postures can lead to bad breathing habits. Being worried, anxious, or scared can affect one, too. Plus, in a quest for flatter abs, many people tend to suck in their stomachs, which forces them to breathe from the chest, not the belly. Not to be forgotten are back or shoulder injuries, which compromise breathing even after they heal. As you just learned, chest-based breathing doesn't use all of the real estate in the lungs; moreover, it keeps you from drawing in the oxygen you need for energy, in order to be productive, to heal, and to sleep well at night.

The goal is straightforward: *Relearn how to breathe moving the breathing back down to the lower part of your body where it belongs.* Okay, maybe getting there is not quite so simple, but when you determine which muscles to use and how to make them as strong as possible, you'll see results quickly. The fact is, the best breathing happens from your chest down. The bottom part of your ribs move, your belly expands, your sides expand, even your back expands.

The exercises in this chapter will help you relearn how to breathe and will strengthen the right muscles so that you'll feel as if you've actually done a workout at the gym. As you practice these exercises, keep in mind that although you should focus on your belly, I don't expect you to continue pushing out your abdomen with every single inhale you take. This is just a way to start reconditioning your body so it will do what it should be doing naturally; the end result won't look or feel as silly as it might at first. Focus on the expansion and contraction of your middle. Both of these movements work your core, so that better breathing will lead naturally to stronger abs and core muscles.

BELLY BREATHING

Belly breathing is the introductory breath that gets you to breathe from the bottom half of your body. When you jut your belly out, you discover the sensation of breathing by using your diaphragm. For a visual, see pages 56–57. Later, much later, you'll be able to expand around the bottom of your ribs without pretending you are Santa Claus.

- Put one hand on your belly and one on your chest, directly under your chin and between your collarbones. Spread your fingers so you can actually gauge movement. Change your breathing so that your top hand does not move at all and your belly expands, almost in an exaggerated way, on the inhale.
- For contrast, do the opposite for a breath or two: have your bottom hand stay still, gaze up, and move your shoulders up on the inhale. Become fully aware of these two very different breaths.

All of this should make sense anatomically. For a visual, see pages 54–55. When you breathe through the lower part of your body (expanding your middle, sides, and back), your diaphragm flattens out and pushes your bottom ribs out. On the exhale, your thoracic diaphragm curls up, emptying your lungs. Again, be patient with yourself; at first it may seem like there are too many pieces of information to juggle. Just keep repeating the belly breathing until it feels totally natural.

Does inhaling and having your middle expand feel completely counter-intuitive? Surprise! You are probably a paradoxical breather (described in Chapter Three). You have been working against your body for years and have, in effect, been taking in a miniscule amount of air compared to what your body needs. This means that when your diaphragm is trying to flatten and pull in more air, expanding your body to add air, you have been "pulling in" and fighting against it.

WARMING UP YOUR DIAPHRAGM

First, tap your sternum with the tips of your fingers to bring your attention to that part of your body. With your pointer fingers right inside the very top, start walking your fingers slowly across the front of your bottom rib. Curve your fingers underneath that rib to bring awareness to the exact place where the diaphragm connects. Imagine in your mind's eye how large this muscle, which traverses your body from side to side, is. While your diaphragm is round and separates the top part of your body from the bottom, it also leans back at your sides and back. Imagine how large your lungs are in the back: they spread to four fingers above your waistline!

Now I want you to go through the exercises that I teach in my class to strengthen all of the muscles involved in perfect respiration.

1. *Alligator.* Lie face down on the floor. Use only your arms to prop up your head and the top of your shoulders. On the inhale, through your mouth, *push the floor away with your belly.* Exhale and flatten out. Remember: Your lower back and butt should not tighten. Number of reps: 10.

2. *Roll Over Alligator.* Place a large book (or a small stack of smaller books) on your abdomen on top of your belly button. (You can use a weight, but books balance better.) While keeping your head flat on the floor, gaze down at the books. Take a belly breath with the goal of making the books rise. As you get better at this exercise, you can graduate to heavier

books or use a 10- or 12-pound weight or kettlebell. If you are advanced and using a heavier weight, focus on letting the weight fall in on the exhale, and seeing how far you can get your bellybutton to go toward your spine. This will make the "push up" that comes with the inhale more challenging. Remember: let the weight push your belly button down toward your spine, and later use this point as a reference to how far you should be able to pull in your stomach. Be careful not to hold your breath in order to push. Number of reps: 10 -15. (When you can do 15, graduate to next weight.)

3. *Cat and Cow.* Roll back over, get on your hands and knees, exhale audibly and round your back up. Hollow out your belly and blow out toward your belly button. On the inhale, just relax your belly and let it expand down with gravity. Notice the rotation in your hips in either position. On the inhale, you form an arch at the bottom of your back, with your tailbone tipped out. On the exhale you rotate your hips forward to create a hollowed-out middle (a C shape).

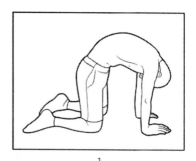

1

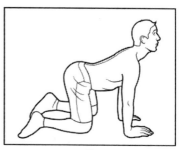

2

Add a Kegel, a pelvic floor contraction,[2] when you exhale, tightening your stomach to empty out all the breath. Remember: your hands should be right under your shoulders. You should not move back and forth; rather you should move up and down. Let your head drop on the exhale, and stretch it up, sipping air above and in front of you on the inhale. On the inhale, focus on really letting go of your stomach, down to the lowest muscles between your hipbones. This is not natural and will take some concentration and practice until you can completely soften this part of your body. Reps: 1 set of 10, then graduate to 2 sets of 10, working your way up to 2 sets of 20. Want to step it up? Hollow your stomach on the exhale, holding it "at the top" for two seconds.

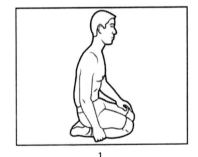

1

4. *Rock and Roll.* Push back so you are sitting up on your knees. You can also be seated in a chair if the floor is uncomfort-

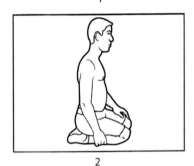

2

---

2. Kegel: an exercise to strengthen your pelvic floor (pubococcygeus) muscles. Both men and women have pelvic floors, comprised of about 20 muscles.

able. On the inhale, move your belly as if you were putting it on your lap, and tilt your lower back away from the back of your chair. You should be creating a curve in the back of your spine. Inhale deeply. On the exhale, lean back as if you were sitting on a couch, pull your stomach in tightly, exhaling hard, and add a Kegel. Make sure you are hollowing out your front on the exhale.

5. *The Perfect Breath.* Change to a standing position and breathe the same way, but now with your arms at your sides. This is best done standing sideways at a full-length mirror. Your shoulders should not move; only your belly and pelvis should be moving back and forth. As you let your belly expand forward, you should be arching your back slightly. This opens up your pelvic floor, so visualize relaxing your pelvic floor and expand your middle. On the exhale, contract your belly, feel your lower abs tighten, tuck in your butt and give a pelvic squeeze in order to push out all the air on your exhale. Now change this exaggerated movement to a subtler one. Make sure you are not in a forward-head posture, and that your ears are directly over your shoulders, spine straight, shoulders back.

Men often have a hard time with the tilt back of the pelvis. The only movement that is similar is when you go to do a squat at the gym, when you arch your lower back and keep your chest up.

What do you achieve with the perfect breath? Well, it:

• Activates your parasympathetic nervous system ("rest and digest").

• Lowers your blood pressure and heart rate.

• Uses the lower, bigger, denser part of the lungs (i.e., is more efficient).

• Helps protect you from constipation, acid reflux, and irritable bowel syndrome.

• Makes for minikegels, so that you avoid pelvic floor problems later in life, such as incontinence, prolapse, and, for women, vulvar pain.

Contrast the perfect breath with the Upper Body Breath (UBB), which does none of these healthy things. In effect, UBB creates pain in your shoulders and neck, raises your blood pressure and anxiety, and brings in much, much less oxygen.

ONE MORE TIME

Do the same exercise you did in the last chapter. When you are on your back, hold a 6-, 8- or 10-pound weight on your stomach (if you feel as if you can handle it, use a small kettlebell). See how far you can let it fall into your stomach. You might want to pick a heavier weight because this is not about raising it, but about seeing how close you can get your bellybutton to your spine. Be careful not to bounce the weight. Sit up, seeing how close you can come to keeping that "bowl" shape while sitting. Stick with it and, after a time, you will be able to maintain that concave bowl shape.

When you are doing Exhale Maximizations, try to mimic the amount of "inward" curve you can get with the weight. Now you are ready to inhale!

INHALE MAXIMIZATIONS

Now that you've cleared out those lungs to make room for more air, it's time to fill 'em up. For a visual, see pages 52–53. Going through the steps below, you will push air into the part of your lungs that have been passive. Keep in mind that most of your lungs are in your sides and back. Divers call this *air-packing*, but they do it more aggressively and with much more experience, so you are only doing a gentle version here—the only one that I recommend.[3] Don't do these exercises on the treadmill or while driving; do them sitting down. And yes, you may feel lightheaded. That's OK; it means you are doing things right.

- Inhale to the max, then sip a little more air at the end. This will fill your alveoli to the fullest rather than just half-full. Note where you feel tightness. Is it by your collarbones, armpits, in your back, where you might have an old injury? Gently stretch these places or use heat to heal and make them more flexible.
- Practice "yogic breath." Fill your belly first, then move your shoulders out to encourage yourself to breathe through the top of your chest and the clavicular area

---

3. Glossopharyngeal inhalation increases the volume of air in the lungs above total lung capacity prior to breath-holding. I'm very familiar with this concept: I worked for Jacques Cousteau in 1988 although I didn't dive at that time in my life.

of your thoracic cavity. Start the breath through your belly, then finish by filling up the top of your lungs. Do this continuously, as if the flow of your breathing mimics a wave.[4] As you become aware of lateral breathing—the expansion of your thoracic cavity from side to side that you feel when you cross your arms in front of you or put your hands in opposite armpits as if keeping them warm—and the expansion of your back when you breathe, this exercise will change subtly.

- At the top of your breath, relax your shoulders and let the air flow into your chest, then soften your pelvis and let yourself sink as if you have let the topmost air go to your middle. This should only take 2 to 3 seconds. Then exhale, *remembering that the exhale is an enthusiastic squeeze.*

As you would with any workout, write down how many reps you do, then, the following day challenge yourself to perform the exercise more strenuously or increase the repetitions.

---

4. Picture in your mind one of those desktop box-like wave machines made of oil and water, and then imagine the flow of your breathing.

EXHALE, INHALE

EXHALE

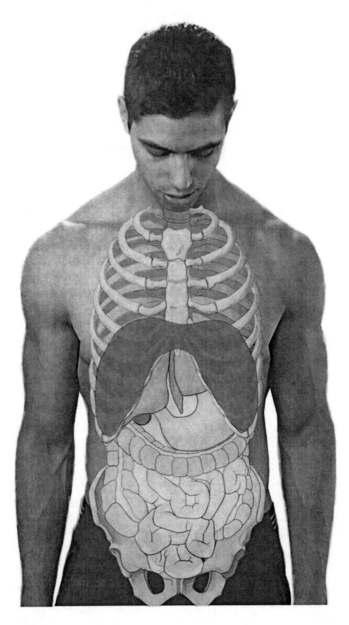

INHALE

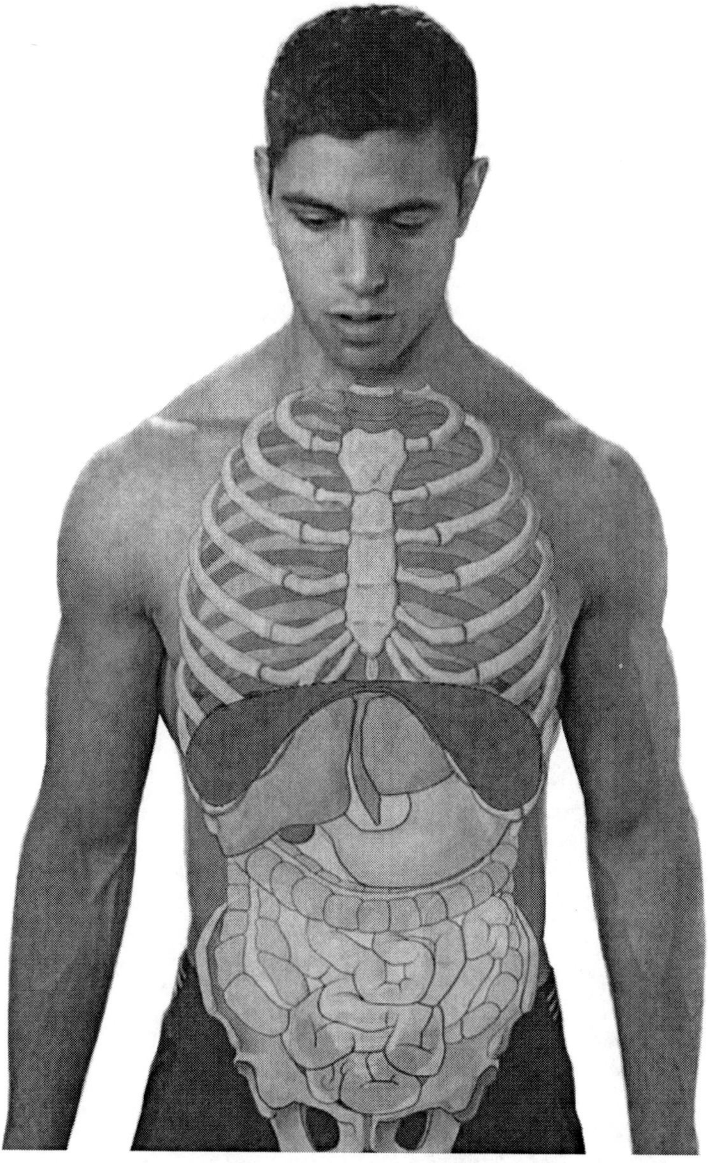

EXHALE

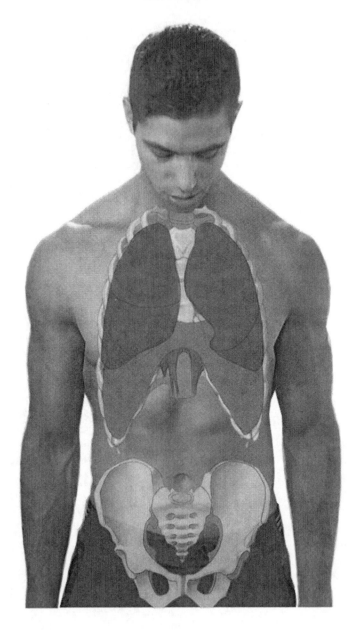

INHALE

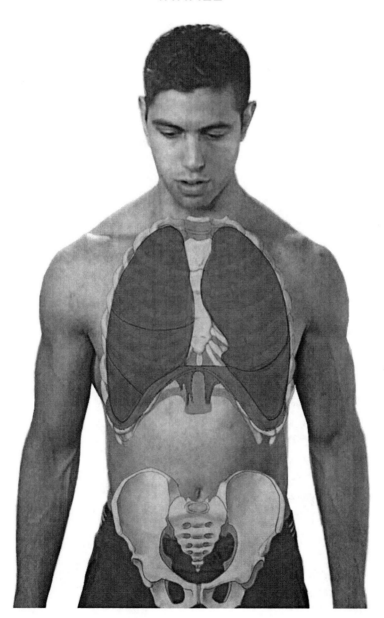

EXHALE

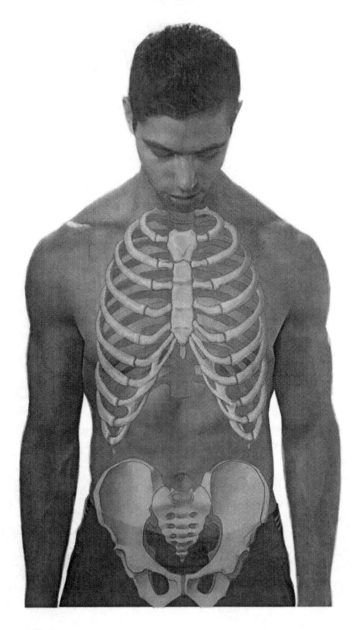

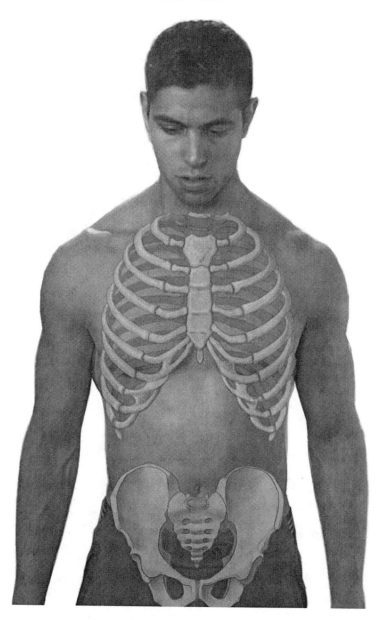

INHALE

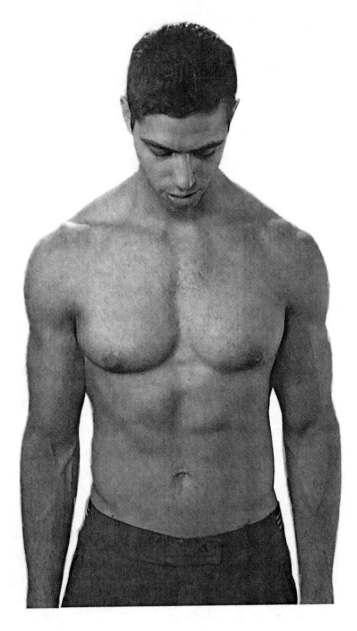

EXHALE

INHALE

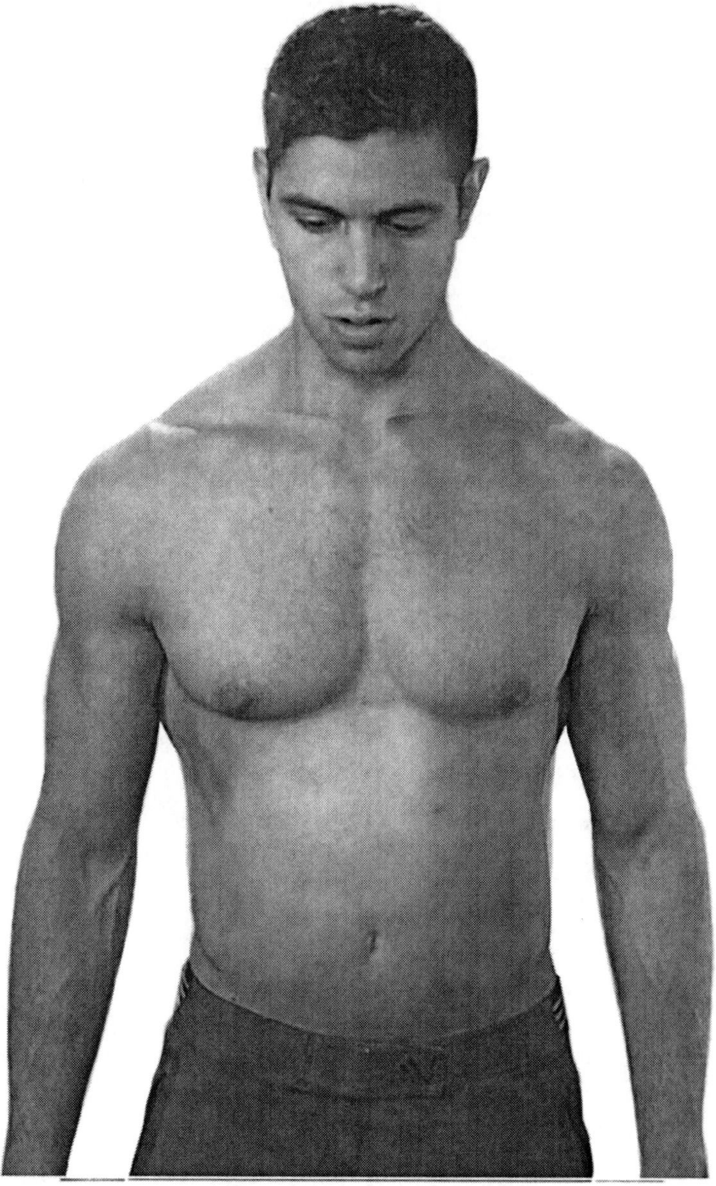

THE WORKOUT

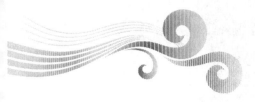

*However intensely you may train, it is
very difficult to strengthen the breathing
muscles because by the time you get them
to the point of overload, you are too tired
to keep up the intensity. You never get to
use that set of "heavier weights" that makes
those specific muscles bigger and stronger.
And cardio? Cardio works your heart, not
your breathing muscles, especially if you
are breathing vertically. The solution? Do
breathing exercises in which only your
breathing muscles are involved.[1]*

DR. BELISA

---

1. Author Allison McConnell explains the need to train breathing muscles
in her book *Breathe Strong, Perform Better:* "the intensity of breathing
work that's needed to hone a person's breathing muscles into optimum
fitness is the same intensity that makes a person so out of breath that the
only option is to stop or slow down—it's a catch 22."

Yes, you definitely can improve your breathing without taxing your heart. And it's not a matter of pumping blood around your body faster; it's about more efficient inhales and exhales.

EXHALE PULSATIONS

Exhale Pulsations are short, sharp exhales that work the muscles involved with exhalation: a pumping action where your abs move from neutral to concave.[2] Your belly "scoops in," even if you have fat around your middle that doesn't naturally "go in." It should feel as if the muscles are pulling your belly button into your body more than ever before. There should be no effort in the inhale; this is an *exhale* exercise.

Determine your baseline. Count how many exhale pulsations you can do in a row. *Be careful: it's easy to continue to blow but not to contract your stomach.* Keep an eye out that you aren't cheating! Note this number.

Exhale Pulsations are easy to do throughout the day since they are inconspicuous. And consider finding a partner. Doing the exercises side by side with someone else can help push you beyond what you might do on your own.

- Beginner level. Exhale through your mouth as if you were blowing out a row of candles, letting the air hit *the back of your teeth* in order to make the exhale

---

2. These are similar to "fire breath" or *kapalbhati* in yoga, a breath that is supposed to purge and clear out your system. According to yoga philosophy, a round of this breath will help you feel less irritable and angry.

audible. If you've never
done this before, it will
help if you put one fin-
ger up at arm's length in
order to feel the exhale.
This is an abs exercise
that targets deeper core
muscles and will enable
you to exhale more effec-
tively. Stronger exhale
muscles and more con-
scious exhaling are very
important because they
make more space in your
lungs for fresh air, and
hence make your inhale

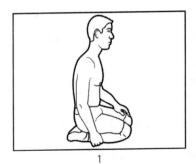

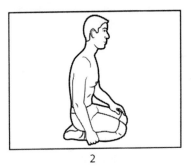

more effective. When you exhale passively, you leave
stale air in your lungs. By strengthening your exhale
muscles, you will unconsciously exhale better. (It's not
as if you have to think about exhaling throughout the
day.)

- Intermediate level. Blow out harder, aiming for a place
  further off in the distance. Make the exhale really
  audible. Exhale harder with the goal of seeing a concave scoop in your middle when you stand sideways
  looking at yourself in a mirror.
- Advanced level. Slow down so that the compression
  feels very intense and you feel a burn sooner. Try pulling your belly button as close to your spine as you

can. Switch to your nose—this automatically makes the inhale and exhale harder since your nostrils are smaller than your mouth.[3]

There are three advanced level variations:

1. Exhale Pulsations in "Table Top" position. Count how many times you can contract, then work on being able to increase that number with time. Use gravity and let your belly really drop, and work on "picking it up."

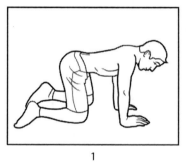
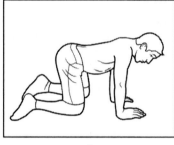

1   2

2. Exhale Pulsations in "Reverse Tabletop" position. Instead of having your back be the top of the table, reverse it and have your belly be the top of the table. Let your head relax back gently. Inhale pushing your belly upwards, and exhale using gravity and letting it fall inward. To move out of this pose, simply lower your butt and raise your head.

3. Exhale Pulsations while retaining. To take it to the next level, you can pulsate *after* you exhale completely, so that no air is coming in or out of your lungs, but your abs are flexing from neutral to concave. Hold your breath (on the exhale) the entire time.

---

3. Want to raise the bar? Do the exhales on an incline (for example, on an inclined sit-up bench).

Your inhale is governed primarily by your diaphragm and intercostal muscles; your exhale is governed by your obliques and other ab muscles. When you learn to recognize which are weaker, you can focus on those areas.

SLOW IT DOWN - BREATHING ISOMETRICS

As in isometrics, slow conscious breathing helps you gain control over your body. Moving a lot of weight with enthusiasm may be good as part of a regular workout, but using your body weight slowly and effectively works specific types of muscles. There are several approaches:

- Exhaling "in steps": let out a little air, then pause with the goal of making your exhale last longer. *Longer* is the goal.
- Counting breaths: there are a few variations of breath-counts. To begin, try the easiest: a four count in, four count out.
- Tactical breathing: this is the one I demonstrate in class, one that is used in the military to induce calm. Inhale six counts, then hold for four counts, exhale for

Q: Will I be sore, like from a regular gym workout?
A: Yes.
Q: I cough and yawn when I do these exercises. Is this normal?
A: Yes, and it's actually good. It means you are pushing yourself and shaking your body out of a normal sedentary breathing state.

six counts, and hold for two. Repeat.

• Coherent Breathing: joins your heartbeat and your breath. Intuitively it makes sense: they should be "talking to" and in line with each other. You want to aim for 5-6 breaths a minute (with heart rate about 60). If you inhale for five seconds and then exhale for five seconds, your body parts are working in unison, in harmony. This type of breathing promotes optimal health and the synchronicity of your body.[4]

These slow breathing isometrics force you to control your muscles over longer periods of time, using "lighter weights." They develop your breathing in a subtler, more important way. They also help lengthen your concentration and focus, *and are in themselves a form of meditation.* If you consider adding a counting breath practice to your routine, the goal should be to do this breathing for a specific length of time—then increase the time as you become more confident of your technique.

THE NEXT 14 DAYS - CREATE A WORKOUT FOR YOURSELF

Get a baseline for yourself for each exercise, even if you are doing just a few reps. Write it down. It has been my experience that there is a crucial learning period for relearning how to breathe: 14 days. Again, as far as your body is con-

---

4. You can read more about "Coherent Breathing" and "Total Breath" in *The Healing Power of the Breath* by Richard Brown and Patricia Gerbarg.

cerned, Lower Body Breath (LBB) is not really a brand new way to breathe; it is one that you used as an infant (even if you don't remember). It also makes sense anatomically: when you inhale, your diaphragm should flatten—hence you are adding anatomical momentum to the learning process. After two weeks of doing these exercises a few minutes a day, they will become natural. You will discover that you are reminding yourself less, and your previous dysfunctional breathing will feel unnatural. For some people this change comes around days 7-10, for others it takes a little longer. It's important that you commit to the 14 days; use whatever method works for you and keeps you on track.

POSTURE

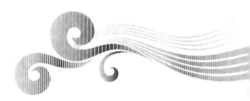

*Oxygenating and balancing your breath
means you are addressing your health
at the root. Not just band-aiding the
symptoms. If you really want 'wellness,'
you need to go back to basics and make
sure the foundation of your health—your
breathing—is good.*

DR. BELISA

Despite being the same person, Superman and Clark Kent adopt very distinct postures. One posture is much like that of a guy who is spending too much time in front of a computer (or in Clark's case, a typewriter): shoulders rounded, neck jutting forward. Along with the thick horn-rimmed glasses and the stutter, this posture portrays a man lacking in confidence. When changing to Superman, Clark removes his glasses, puffs up his chest, and narrows his gaze. Immediately he oozes strength and confidence.[1] Another caricature that depicts a well-known posture is that of Jessica Rabbit. This is a common "selfie" pose for women: butt tilted out, gut sucked in, breasts jutting forward.

Now let's talk about *your* posture. You vacillate between hunched over the wheel or blackberry and a stiff "social" pose. You know your posture is bad but probably have shied away from addressing it because you don't know where to start. Maybe if you ignore it, you hope, it will fix itself or go away, right? Wrong. The bad news is that poor posture is affecting not only your skeleton, it is also impacting the most important thing you do: breathe. The good news is that I am going to give you the Cliff Notes to fix your posture, or at least make it way better.

Consider this: poor posture can affect your ability to breathe by up to 30 percent.[2] Think about that: *30 percent.* That's a third of all the other good work you're doing down the drain. If you're wondering how the position of your

---

1. It's worth checking this link to see the actual drawing of his posture: http://fuckyeahfrankquitely.tumblr.com/image/30262985588

2. Rene Cailliet, M.D., medical author and former director of the Department of Physical Medicine and Rehabilitation at the University of Southern California points out that: ". . . forward head posture (FHP) may result in the loss of 30% of vital lung capacity. These breath-related effects are primarily due to the loss of the cervical lordosis, which blocks the action of the hyoid muscles, especially the inferior hyoid responsible for helping lift the first rib during inhalation." Learn more at: http://zeroto-herotv.com/2012/07/did-you-know-a-forward-head-posture-is-associated-with-a-1-44-greater-rate-of-mortality.

head, neck, shoulders, and back can have such a colossal effect on respiration, the answer is pretty simple: Your head alone is pretty darn heavy. And when your body isn't supporting it as well as it should, the rest of your physical functions get thrown out of whack—big time.[3]

FORWARD HEAD POSTURE (FHP) OR, AS IT'S COLLOQUIALLY CALLED, "TEXT BACK"

Even if your body is in decent shape, it doesn't mean that your breathing is in top form. The same goes for your posture. You can have abs of steel, bulging biceps, and to-die-for delts, but if your skeleton isn't properly aligned, these muscles—as well as your diaphragm, core, and other breathing muscles—aren't working as well as they could or should be.

Do you own a smart phone? Enjoy texting your buddies? Spend a little too much time on Facebook, Instagram, or whatever the latest social media medium is? Are you an office drone at your day job? Spend hours hunched over your laptop? Read a book or your Kindle in your spare time? Got a bad back, bum shoulder, or other injury, new or old? Do you wear a backpack? If you said *yes* to one or more of these questions, then your posture just isn't up to snuff, no matter how hard you're working out at the gym.

---

3. While coming out of the stiff Superman pose may seem easy, it's pretty deeply engrained in us: The study, "It Hurts When I Do This (or You Do That)," published in the *Journal of Experimental Social Psychology,* reported that by simply adopting more dominant poses, people feel more powerful, in control, and able to tolerate more distress.

Yes, your smart phone could be seriously messing with your posture, and that's nothing to LOL at. It's all because of something called Forward Head Position, or FHP. "Text back"—ever heard of it? You will, because FHP is a problem of our modern life and it's not going away anytime soon. FHP occurs when your head is positioned so that your ears are in front of your shoulders instead of directly above them. In other words, your head is forward and down— as if you're still playing that riveting game of Words With Friends—rather than aligned with your neck, shoulders, and back. In comparison, ideal posture means that your head is positioned with your ears over your shoulders, your shoulders are aligned with your pelvis, your pelvis is over your knees, and your knees are over your ankles.

The effects of technology on your posture are hardly exaggerated. Texting places your head an estimated 4.5 inches past your shoulders. And according to chiropractors and other experts, for every inch your head moves forward, *a whopping 10 pounds in weight are added to your upper back and neck muscles.*[4] That's because these muscles have to work much harder to support your head to keep it from dropping onto your chest. It also causes your suboccipital muscles, which support the chin, to be in constant contrac-

---

4. According to Dr. Adalbert Kapandji, for every inch your head moves forwards, it gains 10 pounds in weight as far as the muscles in your upper back and neck are concerned owing to the fact that they have to work that much harder to keep the head (chin) from dropping onto your chest ("A Forward Head Posture Associated With a 1.44 Greater Rate of Mortality and Chronic Back Pain," *Physiology of the Joints*, III). This also forces the suboccipital muscles (they raise the chin) to remain in constant contraction.

tion, which then puts pressure on the related nerves. All told, FHP can add some 30 pounds of work to your cervical spine, throwing your whole skeleton out of alignment.

To get an idea of how this feels, hold a kettlebell directly over your head. Now, bending at the shoulder but keeping your arm straight, hold it at 45 degrees. The weight suddenly feels a lot heavier, doesn't it? Well, this is exactly what happens when you lean your 10-pound noggin forward. Just think of how that can affect your spine and muscles over many years. It's no surprise, then, that FHP can exacerbate old neck, shoulder, and back injuries, too.

Sounds pretty unpleasant, right? But your skeleton and musculature aren't the only things affected by poor posture. In fact, FHP blocks the action of your hyoid muscles, the ones that lift your ribs during inhalation. As a result, you squeeze your lungs and other organs into a cramped position that limits the ability of your diaphragm to do its job. You breathe more shallowly, too. Keep in mind what I said before: you can lose a lot of your lung capacity from FHP, which means that even if you exhale completely and take a big inhale, you still only fill about two-thirds of your lungs with fresh oxygenated air. Plus, poor posture can actually *weaken* your breathing muscles because of all the strain it puts on your body.[5]

---

5. According to research published in the *American Journal of Pain Management,* FHP can also trigger a slew of chronic pain conditions and other health problems, including tension headaches, increased blood pressure, disc herniation, arthritis, pinched nerves, eye and ear dysfunction, fibromyalgia, upper back pain, and reduced shoulder mobility.

If you're still not convinced that your posture is the pits, ask a friend to take a photo of you from the side, both sitting and standing. Take a look: is the back of your head in line with your spine? Or is your head leaning forward, your back curved? Now, make a few adjustments. "Tuck in your ears" by pushing your chin back slightly so that your ears are directly over your shoulders. Take another picture and notice the difference.

IMPROVING YOUR POSTURE: YOUR SHOULDERS

The first step in adjusting and improving your posture is to look at the position of your shoulders. When standing with your back against the wall, your shoulder blades should lie flat against the wall. Be careful not to billow out your chest in order to achieve this. Just slide your shoulder blades together.

Often I see people with rounded shoulders, owing to the fact that their pectoral muscles— the pectoralis major— are constricted (thanks again, computers). Deep tissue massage there can

The postural muscles are there to support you and to maintain the appropriate curve of the spine. The postural muscles of the shoulder include the pectoral muscles (which act internally to rotate the shoulders), the levator scapulae, upper trapezius, scalenes, subscapularis, and suboccipitals. The postural muscles of the trunk include the cervical, thoracic, and lumbar erector spinae muscles. Their job (and to a lesser extent, that of the abdominals) is to extend the spine and keep you erect. In the pelvis and thighs, the postural muscles include the hamstrings, psoas, quads, adductors of the leg, and piriformis.

result in bruising, which is essentially oxygen getting to tissue that wasn't getting it before because it was so constricted. I recommend rolling on tennis balls, then graduating to a Theracane.

IMPROVING YOUR POSTURE: YOUR PELVIS

Now put one hand behind you in order to gauge how much space there is between the curve of your lower back and the wall. There should be just enough to allow you to slide your hand through easily. Too much space? Tilt your pelvis forward to narrow it. Too tight a squeeze? Tilt your butt back so that you create more curve at the back of your spine. Men in general need greater curvature, women need less (but don't worry if you are the exception).

Need help? Tilting your pelvis forward is sometimes a hard concept, so try lying on the floor, and adjusting your hips so that your lower back is pressing into the floor. This is a good way to tilt your pelvis forward. It's the same move when you really slouch into a couch (and find yourself dropping crumbs of whatever you are eating into your

---

Work those pecs. Put your shoulder blades flat on wall. Hard to do? The pectoralis major is the powerful internal rotator of the arm that can cause the shoulders to be pulled down and in towards the chest. Doing external exercises of the arms will decrease the internal rotation of the pectoralis major. Rule of thumb is: when a muscle is 'tight' or increased in tone, work or exercise the opposing muscle; in the case of tight pecs, work the external rotators of the shoulder.

Too often when people think about good posture, about lengthening their spine, they try to stretch upward and consequently pull in their stomachs inadvertently pushing themselves back into dysfunctional Vertical Breathing. Try doing it right: keep yourself belly breathing while reaching upward with the crown of your head. Feels different, right?

bellybutton). Tipping your pelvis back is the position you take when you are about to do a squat at the gym, arching your back.

See if when standing against the wall your back and head are both touching the wall. Making this alignment will feel as if you are leaning back; it is the result of having been leaning forward for so long. In addition to having your head touch the wall, put your hand on the back of your neck to make sure you are creating length. Do this by practicing and experiment by moving your chin down and lengthening your head upwards.

WHAT'S YOUR BRAIN GOT TO DO WITH YOUR POSTURE?

The cerebellum is the part of the brain that controls muscle movement, tone, and, consequently, balance and equilibrium. It also helps control eye movement and is responsible for maintaining postural muscle tone. As I explained earlier, poor posture is due to a weakness in the muscles that maintain good posture. People who have poor posture may suffer from dizziness or orthostatic hypotension (a drop in blood pressure when getting up hurriedly or turning the head quickly), and feel sick when reading in a car. Old injuries, physical inactivity, a career as a desk jockey, and inborn weakness in the nervous system may affect the electrical output of the cerebellum and all that it controls.[6] Physical activity—more specifically exercises that create extension—is the quickest way to improve neurological function and your posture.

Postural weakness and instability may lead to deterioration of spinal joints and eventually degenerative joint disease (severe arthritis) of the spine.[7]

FIX YOUR OWN WORK SETTING ERGONOMICALLY

If you spend at least 35 hours a week in an office, take a serious look at your workspace. Don't wait for new, modern ergonomic furniture to be delivered from high above; *you* can do something about the ergonomics of your work setting.

Your feet should be flat on the ground when sitting; adjust your chair if they are not. When your hands are on the keyboard, the bottom of your arms, wrists or forearms should be parallel to the floor, while your shoulders are relaxed. *Do not move your shoulders up or down in order to get your forearms to the right place.* If you have a laptop, get a separate keyboard. When sitting up straight, examine your viewing angle. You should not be looking up at your

---

6. Weak spinal extension may be the most common culprit, according to Dr. Rob Zembroski.

7. With proper diaphragmatic breathing, the ribs remain low during exhalation and the core stability muscles fire more efficiently, according to Brian Cammarota, athletic trainer at OAA Orthopaedics.

screen; it should be at eye level. The distance should be such that you can read the screen comfortably, without adjustment (e.g., squinting). And if you catch yourself leaning forward to see better, bring the screen in closer, don't you move forward towards it. Make sure you are not leaning forward in an attempt to get your work done faster!

Check your shoulders to make sure they are relaxed and down. Much shoulder pain comes from working at a keyboard that is positioned too high, for which you compensate by raising your shoulders an inch or two. Make sure you relax them and that your desk is accommodating *your* needs. Yes, you may have to move your desk up, add an under-the desk-shelf for your keyboard or a cushion on your chair, but all the changes are worth the effort. *And you definitely are worth it!*

WHY "WORK HARD, PLAY HARD" IS HURTING YOU

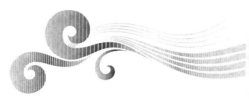

Check your breathing when you are listening to a disturbing news story. Whereas you are nowhere near the event and might never have experienced that trauma, your body tightens and your breathing gets shallow. Worrying has the same effect on your body: it tenses, as if getting ready for a challenge. All this takes energy from your body; all this makes your breathing shallower. Imagine the effect after hours, days or weeks of living this way. It is time to change that in order to have more energy, to oxygenate and relax your body, to take better care of it.

DR. BELISA

"WHAT DOESN'T KILL YOU WILL MAKE YOU STRONGER" NO LONGER APPLIES

You complain that you are stressed-out, that you are tired, that you need to relax, but these proclamations are rhetorical. The person next to you probably agrees that they are, too. You share stories and commiserate with friends on the fact that you don't get enough sleep and that you are exhausted. The people you talk to may rotate, depending on the day, but the script is the same. And everyone agrees: your hairdresser, coworker, neighbor, best friend. But now I am putting you on notice: you've been saying the same things for months, even years. Time to address it.

To add to the problem, our society glorifies busy.[1] The busy person appears important, and multitasking is something you almost feel a competitive urge to get better at. Then you stress out. The solutions are temporary: massage, a bath, a couple drinks. Or sometimes you just wait it out until your next vacation, or you simply chalk it up to the fact that life will not change because this is just how modern life is. Stressful.

Which brings us to the adage "What can't kill you will only make you stronger."[2] Right? Wrong. The impact of

---

1. See a recent ad in which a utility company proudly announces that it, too, is "on" 24/7, as are its customers: http://www.coned.com/customercentral/PDF/everything-matters/You%20Dont%20Have%20an%20Off%20Switch%20Why%20Should%20We.pdf.

2. The saying, "What doesn't kill me makes me stronger," appears in Nietzsche's *Twilight of the Idols*. While pushing yourself to tolerate more chronic stress will not inoculate you against it, stressful events may make

stress can take years off your lifespan, and even if it doesn't, it does diminish the quality of life. Several sources report that workplace stress costs U.S. employers an estimated $200 billion per year, and many stress-related illnesses can turn into major medical problems.

Some folks find the impact of stress on their lives hard to believe. They look around, saying, I feel as stressed out as everyone else, then they shrug it off. Well, yes, society has in effect convinced people that lack of sleep is normal, that not being able to turn off the chatter when they try to fall asleep is normal, and that lying in bed watching news, writing texts or doing quasi-social things like responding to a Facebook post keeps them current. And then there are the beeping, honking, and buzzing appliances that require immediate attention.

Each year you make some kind of formal or informal pact with yourself that you will prioritize better. Relax more, stress less. Take care of yourself. Carve out more "me time" in your non-stop schedule. And each year this resolution lasts between 48 hours and a week at most, until you stop trying to meditate, keep a journal, take walks, be in "the now," and just go back to what is easiest—being stressed out.

---

you a stronger person. Malcolm Gladwell's latest book, *David and Goliath*, examines the relationship between "remote misses" and extraordinary achievement, and how difficult childhoods can foster strength and lead to life of outstanding accomplishments—another way of saying that "what doesn't kill you makes you stronger."

So how much stress is in fact brought on by you? How much does stress actually drive you? Are you one of those people who did best in school by cramming and writing papers the night before? Do you feel pride in getting more done today than yesterday? If so, then you do have some of the stress-addict in you, and given that you may not be healing from whatever ails you as fast as you want, or not be healing at all given that you are succumbing to another one of the common ailments that have to do with stress (e.g., acid reflux, trouble sleeping, fatigue, and anxiety), you may want to reevaluate your perceptions of stress so you can make some real changes.

Your body and mind can tolerate a certain amount of stress, as long as there is an adequate amount of downtime to rest and recharge. Watching "brainless TV" or spending time on Facebook is not really time out. In fact, for many people, just sitting still without any kind of input (music, background TV, etc.) has become hard to do.

QUIZ: ARE YOU A STRESS ADDICT?

If part of you likes and strives under stress,[3] and part of you knows it's hurting you and is trying to find peace and bal-

---

3. According to research in the field, "While stress is often associated with negative affect and distress, it can include 'good stress' which is based on external and internal stimuli that are mild or moderately challenging but limited in duration and results in cognitive and behavioral responses that generate a sense of mastery and accomplishment, and can be perceived as pleasant and exciting" (*Annals of the NY Academy of Sciences*, 2008).

ance, the addicted side, the one with the strength of years of habit, is going to win. To start to make a change, you need more insight, and a good place to start is by noting which of the following behaviors resonates with you. These are the top ten patterns that define a stress addict.

1. You feel pride in having completed an imposing daily to-do list. Whether it makes you feel like supermom or just genetically superior to your friends, there is smugness underneath the complaining.[4]

2. You get a rush from running. Whether it's running to the supermarket, the drycleaners or the gym, the pressure of coordinating tasks and achieving goals gives you a rush.

3. You get excited about the idea of multi-tasking and thereby being more efficient. You want to pat yourself on the back when you are able to do four things well at the same time (which also leads to love of gadgets that profess to help you multitask better).

4. You feel important. The idea that so many people need you and that your contribution is essential leads you to feel wanted and useful. Just think of the chaos if you weren't around.

5. You feel strong and in control because you can tolerate pressure and you take pride in not being lazy. At the same time, you get irritated at people for being so slow and getting in your way when you are on a manic roll.

---

4. The Navy SEALS are trained to be "comfortable in chaos" in order to meet unbelievable challenges, but you have not received that training.

6. Deep down inside you believe that stress-related problems are really genetic or accident-related.

7. You feel uncomfortable, worried, and nervous when you don't have something you must do right away. And what you "need" to do becomes absolute.

8. You depend on and look forward to the buzz of a caffeine high, and at times wish you could survive on less sleep or take a food pill instead of "wasting time" eating and sleeping.

9. You thrive on taking short cuts and closing the deal, meeting the deadline. You find yourself saying (or thinking) "get to the point!" more and more often.

10. You find it difficult to be in the present. You are always either planning for the future or mulling about something in the past. When looking at time, it seems to have flown by.

If any one of these behaviors rings a bell,[5] it's time for you to change your life style because it is part of a larger pattern of stress addiction. That's the bad news. Now the good news is that if you have gotten this far in this book, you can make a big change in your life. Read on!

---

5. Dr. Peter Whybrow, director of the Institute for Neuroscience and Human Behavior at UCLA, explores the rise of stress addiction and the consequences of what he calls "the symptoms of clinical mania" in his forthcoming book, *The Intuitive Mind: Common Sense for the Common Good.* Two *New York Times* articles, written five years apart, discuss why hypomania is so attractive to the person experiencing it in the workplace. http://www.nytimes.com/2010/09/19/business/19entre.html?pagewanted=all&_r=0 http://www.nytimes.com/2005/03/22/health/psychology/22hypo.html

RANK YOUR STRESS

- Stress yellow: You are starting to have trouble sleeping because you can't turn off "the chatter." You might have been told that you grind your teeth at night. You think about work long after the day is done. You find yourself grasping for strategies to help manage whatever it is you have to do. The weekend passes away too quickly and there never seems to be enough "me time." You remember a time when you were less stressed and maybe happier. You are taking less care of yourself simply because there aren't enough hours in the day.

- Stress orange: All the characteristics of yellow have become the norm. Plus now you find yourself irritable, and occasionally experience disturbing episodes such as road rage when you lose control. You snap at people you love, then feel intense guilt. You are often angry with yourself for not getting everything done. You fantasize about vacations or just getting up and leaving town. These fantasies are replaced by those in which you go postal. You are taking medications

---

What happens when you experience stress? Powerful hormones are released throughout the body, elevating blood pressure and putting the senses on high alert. Glucose is driven up to the brain and into the muscles. Your evolutionary preprogrammed response is fight or flight. You are probably in a mild to moderate state of fight to flight all the time, as a "normal" thing—but it definitely is not normal.

---

to sleep and are drinking way too much caffeine or energy drinks in order to be alert during the day.

- Stress red: You have been diagnosed with medical problems that are stress-related (e.g., ulcer or migraine). You have been told by your doctor that as part of your recovery you must address the stress in your life or you can expect your health problems to be chronic, and that they will affect your quality of life/lifespan. Your mental or physical health has been impacted by stress, which could be related to your worry over future stress, your trauma of past stress, or your subjective perception of your current stress. You have been diagnosed with an anxiety or depressive disorder, and therapy and/or medications have been recommended. While anxiety or depressive disorders can have physiological bases, stress can significantly worsen both.

If you stay at level yellow for more than a year, orange for more than a few months, or red for more than a few weeks, there can be serious physical and mental health consequences. The number of injuries you will suffer—because you didn't notice an important detail or were distracted—may increase. Self-medicating incidents will augment. Your body's immune system runs amok because stress disrupts the body's ability to heal itself. The time spent on going to appointments or money on medications (usually pain medications) will increase.

You may find yourself feeling distanced from and irritated by your spouse, and your relationships with colleagues and supervisors may feel strained. You may find yourself relying more on alcohol or shopping to relax. And ultimately, you'll find yourself living less in the present. You'll be nostalgic about a "simple" past you once had, or dream about the more balanced life you hope to have in the future. You may get forgetful because stress affects the hippocampus in the brain, so that it is hard to remember things you once knew perfectly well. Days and months will whiz by.

> Women experience stress with greater intensity than men. They process words and body language more quickly by using both sides of the brain (which predisposes them to multi-tasking), and have a deeper limbic system, the seat of emotions (which connects one more sensitively to all relationships).

STRESS MAKES YOU FAT
(AND FAT MAKES YOU STRESSED)

Did you know that stress gives you belly fat? (Even baboons get muffin tops when they are stressed-out in the wild!) If you are trying to lose weight, stress very well might be the reason for the plateau in your diet.

Yes, you and your best friend may both be following a new diet, yet your friend will be losing pounds and you will slowly, painfully, be losing ounces. Then you hit that dreaded plateau of eat less, work out more, and stay at the same weight. Sound familiar? The one factor you haven't taken into account is your *cortisol level.* If you have a higher level of stress hormone in your body than she does, it's going

Breathing exercises can become a tremendous source of support in your losing weight. They can help you gain body awareness and consequently deal with cravings and impulse eating. Breathing exercises can help you feel satiated, and thus be instrumental in helping you develop healthier eating habits. Keep track of your cravings and how the breathing exercises minimize them.

to be harder for you to lose weight.[6] That "stress weight" tends to accumulate and stick like glue to your middle. You may look objectively at both your lives and try to analyze who has more stress, and try to figure out the different ways you both handle it. For example, you worry. She, not so much. Your body doesn't distinguish between fear or anxiety about possible things in the future and your fear of a real threat that is happening today.[7]

THE ULTIMATE STRESS SOLUTION: BREATHING

Which came first: the anxious, shallow Upper Body Breathing (vertical) or the stress? Regardless, you are in the loop. Breathing badly you feel stressed, the stress then pushes you to breathe worse—you take shallow, erratic, small breaths. This in turn alerts your nervous system to go deeper into

6. *Why Zebras Don't Get Ulcers* by Robert Sapolsky explores other fascinating effects of stress. The PBS special, "Stress: Portrait of a Killer," highlights his research, which was conducted on baboons in Africa. It is viewable on YouTube: http://www.youtube.com/watch?v=eYG0ZuTv5rs.

7. Can breathing and meditation help? You betcha:
http://www.ncbi.nlm.nih.gov/pubmed/23527522
http://www.ncbi.nlm.nih.gov/pmc/articles/PMC3184496/.

fight or flight, which then constricts your breath even more. Are you in a warzone? Nope, just crouched over your computer, growing more impatient and full of anxiety with every hour, stressed about your to-do list, your project deadline, and all the things that demand your immediate attention.

Changing the way you breathe will lower stress levels within minutes. Faster than a Valium, a double shot of scotch, or a good massage. Yes, you yourself can lower your blood pressure faster (and with less side effects) than any medication. If you could hook yourself up to a machine that measures galvanic skin response, heart rate, blood pressure, and brain waves within seconds, all the signs that your body is calming would show up on a screen. Sometimes it's hard to believe that changing the way that you breathe works without your being attached to machines that measure your body response quantitatively.

Find a way to quantify your stress at the moment, then do your exercises, and finally "measure" (whatever your way to measure is), and see the change. Several of my patients have attested to the efficacy of breathing efficiently:

> "My measure of my anxiety was when I could feel
> my heart beat. When I am about to have a panic
> attack it rises to my throat and I have trouble
> focusing on anything else, my vision for things far
> away and in the periphery gets short. My hands
> get cold and sweat. When all these come together,
> I know a full-blown panic attack is on the way. So
> I made that my measure: the next few times that

happened, I put on my earphones and listened to
the breath count. I timed how long it took me to
feel my heart go back down. I realized that I had
a moment of "turning the corner" when I would
think, 'I'm going to be ok,' and the escalating
would stop. For the next 14 days I practiced
'bringing myself down'—it was fascinating to me
that it worked every single time. Then it got to be
how fast I could bring myself down. How, when I
get a hint of anxiety, I do a few deep LBB breaths
to 'reset' myself and keep moving."

"On Sunday night, I'd lie in bed trying to get to
sleep but my brain would not be able to turn off.
I'd run through scenarios, to-do lists, everything
about the week ahead of me. As time went by,
I'd get more upset at what was left of the night
for me to sleep, knowing for sure I'd now be
starting Monday tired. Relearning how to breathe
and oxygenating myself better during the day,
then having a relaxing breathing practice for
before getting into bed meant that rarely happens
anymore."

THE SOLUTION: RECOVERY BREATH

You do not have to take a meditation class in India or
undergo long-term psychoanalytic therapy in order to learn
to live in the now. Short "active meditation" breathing techniques can lower your blood pressure, heart rate, and cor-

tisol levels when practiced a few minutes a day. This daily "reboot" is exactly what you need. You don't need a vacation, you don't have to bear down and plow through work, day after day, without rest until you get to your next vacation; you just need to *turn stress off* at regular intervals. You need to "turn off" so that your immune system can recharge—and you are about to learn how to do this with Recovery Breath. Recovery Breath is an active meditation that is a culmination of all the exercises detailed in previous chapters. It is a gentle version of what is done in class, under my supervision, and it is explained in the next chapter.

MEDITATION FOR PEOPLE WHO CAN'T MEDITATE

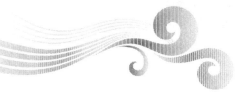

*What if I said I had a medicine that would
keep you calm, but alert? That would
relax and energize you. That would help
you recover, boost your immune system,
lower the oxidative stress that causes aging,
power you up and fuel every cell in your
body from your frazzled brain to your
taxed muscles. You'd say, "Give it to me,"
right? Well, here it is. And no side effects.
Take it every day—doctor's orders.*

DR. BELISA

Recovery Breath is a form of active meditation and is completely different from any perception you have of meditation. It's called *Recovery Breath* because it is a two-part breathing exercise that helps reset your body after undergoing a grueling day at work, a disagreement with your spouse, a test or competition—any taxing or demanding situation.

If your usual routine during the week is to push hard and keep yourself going full speed until you get to the weekend, the best thing you can do is practice Recovery Breath five minutes a day. Yes, only five minutes a day! It won't make you groggy; in fact, if anything, it will refuel you. It will drench your body and every cell in it with oxygen, which is a big relief in view of the fact that your body has been running on unbalanced levels of carbon dioxide and low oxygen, adrenaline, caffeine, and pressure owing to your hectic schedule.

So, you may ask, after those five minutes, can I just hop back into my stressful existence and keep on going? Yes, indeed you can; but you'll have increased mental clarity and more energy, and actually be able to problem-solve better and handle any irritability and stress you encounter during the day.

Long term, you'll protect yourself against high cortisol, heart disease, back problems, and migraines—and a host of diseases caused by chronic stress.

HEAR YOURSELF THINK

Your first question probably is, what specifically will this type of breathing/meditation do for me? I'll answer that succinctly. It will:

1. Quiet your mind so you can hear yourself think.

2. Let you distance yourself from your past so that you can live more in the present. This is what mindfulness is.
3. Calm you to the point that you can hear your inner voice, be guided by your intuition.
4. Make you feel centered, balanced and give you a distinct awareness of "your core."
5. Make you feel more connected to your own feelings, and to those of others.

HOW LONG DO I DO THE TWO-PART BREATH?

Initially, you will aim to do the two-part breath for two minutes; later you may graduate to three or four. To begin, set a gentle alarm to signal two minutes or find a song that you can have playing in the background for that time period. Since you are not doing this exercise with a guided breathwork practitioner, it will be gentler than the one you would do if you were in an actual class. The reason for this is that since breathing is both a conscious and unconscious process, it bridges both parts of your brain. Some people may have a cathartic[1] response or release, and if they have suffered trauma in the past that they are now addressing, it is advisable to have someone to guide them through the exercise. If you are dealing with minimal routine stress and augment the time or difficulty of the two-part breath slowly each time you do it, there won't be an issue.

---

1. Adjective derived from 'catharsis,' originally referring to purging but now commonly used to describe the feeling of relief that follows the expression of emotional tensions.

Feel like shedding a tear, smiling or laughing during this exercise? It is normal; it is a cathartic response. If this happens to you, don't repress the feeling. Let it out. Even if you don't know why it's happening, you'll undoubtedly feel lighter later.

INSTRUCTIONS FOR THE RECOVERY BREATH: PART ONE

The two-part breath starts with two inhales. The first inhale fills your belly, the second, the top of your lungs. There is a very distinct division between the first and the second inhale, and each one should sound slightly different. The first one (which is a LBB) is fuller as well.

1. Lying on your back, with nothing under your head, put one hand on your belly and one on the top of your chest, by your collarbones.

2. Breathe through your mouth. It is a bigger orifice than your nostrils, and the point of this exercise is to get more oxygen into your body and accustom yourself to breathing this way for this exercise. It may feel peculiar at first, but you will get used to it after the second or third time.

3. The first inhale should make your belly rise; your top hand (on your chest) should not move. Now, without exhaling, take another inhale and fill the top of your lungs. This time your top hand should move. To help you "learn" the breath, you can move your shoulders

back slightly. *Be sure that you are not just transferring air from the bottom to the top.*

4. There should be two distinct inhales, even if the second one is small. It is not one long breath. Your belly should remain full as you add the second "top" breath. The first few times you inhale this way may feel odd. It should; you've never breathed like this before.

5. Exhale, making sure that your exhale is dynamic: it should take the amount of time the two inhales took, not longer. Exhale in one breath, feeling your chest and belly contract.

This first part in Recovery Breath *should* be hard; it is *exercise* for your breathing muscles. Note that the second inhale will feel smaller, even more constricted. You will probably feel pressure around your collarbones or armpits as you try to fill up this second breath. Some people even experience a "stitch" in their back as they try this new breathing, others a tightness in their necks. The general rule is to relax that place and continue inhaling.

Your ego and your body may struggle with the newness of this exercise. Watch your reaction. Is it one of curiosity or irritation? Is it to react immediately, not to like what you are doing, even to judge it, or are you able to remain open-minded and gentle with your exercise?

There are three things to remember during this exercise:

1. Keep breathing through your mouth for the entire first part. You may switch to your nose for the second part.

2. Find a rhythm that suits you, and stick to it. You should

be able to find or "drop down" into this rhythm with more ease each time.

3. No matter what happens, just calmly and firmly encourage yourself to continue breathing. Any peculiar or uncomfortable sensations will lessen each time you practice, and the benefits are priceless.

It may help you to read the initial reactions of some of my patients:

I immediately got lightheaded as I did the two-part breath, but since I was lying down, all I had to do was remind myself that I couldn't fall so it was safe. The feeling of newness was hard to deal with . . . as an adult we almost never experience anything totally new where we have to trust that is good for us (like when I was a kid). Though I would see myself hesitate, I just kept encouraging myself to continue. The first time was the hardest. After that I think my breathing muscles got stronger and my understanding of the benefits outweighed my being skeptical and even a bit afraid. Afterwards I felt lighter and recharged, like I'd taken a great nap.

Falling into a rhythm was what I focused on. I listened to my own breathing and just kept telling myself to keep with it, just as when I am running. I hit a wall, but struggled through it and got a "second wind." It was oddly difficult given that I was lying on my back. For part of the time I was

just confused as to why it was so hard. I had to
shut out the talk in my head that wanted me to
stop. I just told myself that I had nothing to lose
and that it wasn't frightening . . . it was interesting.
Knowing that I was super-oxygenating my body
and working out my breathing muscles made it
easier to push through that hard moment, and
though the subsequent times I practiced it was still
work, it wasn't as hard as the first time.

Understand that you will hit a wall. Some people hit it after 20 breaths, others significantly later. In fact, the first few times you practice this active meditation you will hit the same kind of wall that you do when you work out. You will hear yourself make excuses about how you want to stop. Treat this feeling just as you do any other time you don't want to continue doing something but have to. If you feel a little tingling, that's OK! Just encourage yourself to keep going, remind yourself you are doing well and are almost done. Believe that there will be a moment when you get "to the other side," and just keep moving to the pace of your breath. It won't be like trudging uphill anymore.

INSTRUCTIONS FOR THE RECOVERY BREATH: PART TWO

Now you are going to switch to a big, gentle inhale and a big, gentle exhale.

1. Move your hands away from your body. Put your arms at your sides, palms up. Point your toes away

from each other. You may keep breathing through your mouth or switch to your nose. Relax your lips, your face, your palate (the roof of your mouth). Let your tongue get heavy. Very important: let your jaw relax. All of your body takes cues from your jaw. Pay attention to your cheeks, ears and neck, relaxing them with each exhale. Relax your shoulders and your whole body—all the way to the tips of your fingers.

2. Continue doing body scans from time to time to make sure you are not holding tension anywhere. You will be surprised to discover that you may have a place that is always tensed, so much so that you have become accustomed to it. Really sense that with each inhale you are letting yourself float a little higher, and with each exhale you are letting yourself sink a little deeper. Try to move your mind away from thinking, and just keep your attention on physical sensations, then on watching. By "watching" I mean watch your body breathe as if you were watching another person.

Recovery Breath is pithy, involves active participation, and is immediately rewarding. It is a "two-for the price-of one" bargain: a brief but highly effective exercise that helps you recover from one day to the next, a form of active meditation for people who "can't meditate." By relaxing your body so that stress hormones and blood pressure decrease, it recharges your battery within minutes and encourages mindfulness. It protects you against the effects of prolonged stress by giving your body the oxygen and relaxation it needs to recover. In addition, it is a breathing exercise that you can taper to meet your needs and level of enthusiasm.[2]

In sum, Recovery Breath is a "reset" that will give your immune system a boost, keep your cortisol and blood pressure down, and oxygenate your body so that oxidative stress doesn't age you before your time. Do it as often as possible, ideally every day.

---

2. Are you liking the spiritual part of this more than you thought? Consider reading David Elliot's *Healing* or Judith Kravitz' *Breathe Deep Laugh Loudly*; listening to Jack Kornfield's YouTube discussions or Dharma Punx' podcasts; or ordering authors like Pema Chodron or Thich Nhat Hanh from Sounds True, Inc.

BREATHING FOR CHILDREN

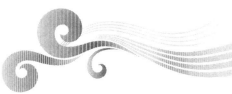

*Gen Z (the "post-millennials") is going
to be faced with serious health problems
owing to their growing up in an instant-
access techie world. Hunched over tiny
screens that impose limited eye movement,
their posture is unhealthy; and physical
movements are limited to clicks or swipes
of their fingers. Without a change in our
children's lifestyle, the result will be an
eventual narrowing of their intrapsychic
and interpersonal awareness and lower
intakes of oxygen than generations before.*

DR. BELISA

For a parent, caretaker or teacher, the ideal way to teach a
child a new skill or behavior is to model it. Consequently,
if you are a dysfunctional breather, your child could mimic

Use breathing to help children understand how important intuition is and how to determine where their core is. Listening to their own breathing can teach them the importance of quiet, of being still. In teaching children how to stay safe, listening to their "gut" is the best protection you can give them. This is only possible if they learn to pause, listen to their inner voice, and look at detail. They will also recognize feelings of discomfort or alarm within themselves.

---

your breathing, thereby picking up your bad habits. However, you *can* change this and influence how your children feel and function simply by changing the way that you and, accordingly, they breathe.

When children become anxious or fearful, their breath becomes short and shallow. As in adults, their sympathetic nervous system responds as if there were an emergency and prepares for "fight or flight." The chemical-electrical impulses that allow for communication between the limbic system and the neocortex become so overwhelmed that communication shuts down.[1] As a result, it is difficult for them to think clearly or make decisions, and learning can become impaired.

HAVE CHILDREN PRACTICE LBB

1. Emphasize that a deep breath does not mean raising the shoulders; it means widening in the middle. (Ask any ten-year-old to take a deep breath and observe

---

1. The neocortex is the portion of the brain involved in higher order thinking skills, such as analysis and evaluation, conscious thought, and reasoning.

how they have already assimilated UBB by raising their shoulders to their ears). When you take a deep breath, put your hand on your own stomach. Have your child do the same.

2. Stress that the breath helps them pause and think. Pairing a physical task with instructions to stop and pause makes for ease in learning. This approach can change in sophistication as you evolve into talking about mindfulness, compassion, and impulse control. These three topics have become especially important as we see Gen Z encounter more problems with frustration tolerance, narcissism, entitlement, reality testing, and judgment.

3. Take advantage of game or game-like activities that focus on breathing and that appeal to children. Explain to them how this ability to focus has tremendous benefits. Have children blow through a straw or on an imaginary cup of hot cocoa or bowl of soup as a way to regulate and pace themselves.

USING GAMES TO FOSTER GOOD BREATHING HABITS

There are several important modifications to keep in mind when using games to teach children:

1. Time: keep the time they "play" short. For very young children this may mean as little as ten seconds.

2. Reward: make sure that there is concrete, positive reinforcement that is age-appropriate. For younger children, being able to play video games later on in

the evening as a reward is too abstract. Give them a quarter, a piece of gum, a gold star at the end of the exercise.

3. Exhale tools: use anything round that moves. I've used little pom-poms from the craft store. Set up a line and have your child blow each one across the line.

4. Remember that for children the goal isn't lung expansion as much as it is about body awareness, good exhales, and "slowing down."

Use the breathing techniques with children before exams, sporting competitions, performances, etc., to foster confidence and a sense of calm.

BREATHING EXERCISES FOR CHILDREN

- Inhales: have them breathe in unison with you, pushing their belly out with the inhale. Lying down helps them concentrate a bit better. Starting with 5 inhales is a good idea.

- Exhales: also do the exhale pulsations together. Make sure to give the child a star or prize after a set number, 10, 15, or 20. If you have two kids, one can count and the other one can blow. Remember to teach them that on the exhale they are "emptying the balloon," meaning their stomach contracts. (Blowing up pre-stretched balloons is an addition to this exercise.)

Keep in mind that children breathe faster than adults. Infants can breathe up to 60 breaths per minute; children up to age five, 20-30 breaths a minute; and up to age 12, 12-20 breaths a minute.

- Slow exhales: get your children to watch the seconds hand on a clock. Having them try to lengthen the amount of time they exhale will encourage better emotional and breathing control. Again, the goal is not to get them to hold their breath in times of stress; rather it is to have them strive to maintain a continual deep flow, and to slow down expiration.
- The counting breath (4, 4, 6, 2): this exercise is a good one to finish up with. Have them close their eyes and breathe through their nose. This is one that can become a ritual to get them to sleep (or to help them get back to sleep after an interruption).

Remember that belly breathing will automatically get children to calm down. Lower Body Breathing is connected to the parasympathetic nervous system, which means that coaching and modeling LBB will ultimately teach them how to calm themselves down.

LBB AND CHILDREN WITH SPECIAL NEEDS

Breathing exercises for children can be particularly beneficial for those with special needs because it can help to avoid panic, aggression, meltdowns, or tantrums. Often games

Could childhood sleep problems lead to behavioral problems? Research says *yes:* decreased sleep in children has led to attention-deficit/hyperactivity disorder (ADHD)-like behavior problems.[2] Another study reports that approximately ten per cent of 6-8 year olds have sleep-disordered breathing.[3] The risk is increased among children with enlarged tonsils, cross-bite, and convex facial profile.

found online will ask them to imagine that there is a balloon in their belly, thus encouraging Lower Body Breath. There are several sites that help children focus by breathing.[4] You might consider buying attractive yoga mats that are made for children. Setting aside a time for these exercises could include fetching the mat and putting it away at the end of the session. Always keep in mind the recommended modifications for children when undertaking these exercises.

- Shooting stars breathing exercise. Children inhale as they raise their hands above their heads, and exhale as they lower them, wiggling their fingers.
- Blowing bubbles, blowing on a pinwheel, a feather.

2. A study conduced at the University of Helsinki and the National Institute of Health and Welfare, Finland, in 2009, with over 200 children.

3. Over 500 children were involved in a study led by the Institute of Biomedicine at the University of Eastern Finland. The results were published in the European Journal of Pediatrics.

4.   http://video.about.com/kidsactivities/Breathing-Exercises-to-Help-Children-Relax.htm; also practicing different breaths related to animals, hissing or smelling flowers (http://move-with-me.com/self-regulation/4-breathing-exercises-for-kids-to-empower-calm-and-self-regulate/)

In this exercise, make sure the children also focus on the inhales. Set times for maintaining the breaths, and establish an age-appropriate pace.

• Bhramari pranayama or the "bee breath" takes its name from the word for the black Indian bumblebee, bhramari. The adjective bhramarin is Sanskrit for "sweet as honey." Have your child practice making that sound: inhale through your nose and exhale a soft sound like the buzzing of a bee.

A FEW MORE TIPS

1. Often covering your children's ears or having them wear earplugs in a noisy setting will help them focus internally rather than externally. If your child likes a particular tune with a steady rhythm, you might have it as background music.

2. Practice when your child is calm and receptive; don't wait for a crisis—a tantrum or a meltdown—to introduce a breathing exercise.

3. Use examples that make sense to them, not you. Good illustrations are available on the sites referenced. Be willing to demonstrate the exercise several times before having the child join you.

4. Be patient. More often than not, it will take a child several attempts to feel the difference in patterns—and don't forget the rewards!

GLOSSARY OF TYPES OF BREATHING

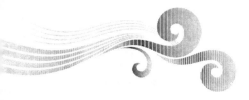

This list is not exhaustive; these are breathing exercises and methods that you may research and consider now that you have a good foundation for basic breathing.

BELLY BREATHING: Also known as Abdominal or Diaphragmatic Breathing, it is marked by expansion of the abdomen rather than the chest, and encourages full oxygen exchange. By contracting the diaphragm, a muscle located horizontally between the chest cavity and stomach cavity, air enters the lungs and the belly.

BREATHWALK: Combines distinct patterns of breathing—ratios, intervals and breath types—that are synchronized with walking steps and meditative attention. Directed breathing and focused attention can be utilized for personal growth, to control pain, and to induce relaxation, and are used by many forms of martial arts and athletics. Some examples of patterns are: The Hawk, Dove, Blissful Eagle, and Magnificent Lion.

BUDDHIST BREATHING: Buddha quite openly and continually advocated Breath Meditation or *Anapanasati*, an awareness of the inhaling and exhaling breaths. It starts with an awareness of the ordinary physical breath, which, when cultivated correctly, leads into higher awareness. By centering one's senses on the activity of breathing, this heightened awareness focuses on the areas of the abdomen and the chest and the expanding and contracting of the belly, and leads to "self-reporting" of movements.

BUTEYKO BREATHING: Based on the assumption that numerous medical conditions, especially asthma, are caused by hyperventilation, this breathing technique (breathe slowly through the nose) was developed in the 1950s by Konstantin Buteyko, a Ukrainian doctor. It purports to break the vicious cycle of rapid, gasping breaths, airway constriction and wheezing.

CIRCULAR BREATH: Produces a continuous tone, often used by players of wind instruments. By breathing *in* through the nose while simultaneously pushing air *out* through the mouth using air stored in the cheeks, an uninterrupted tone is achieved. It is used extensively in playing many instruments; e.g., the Australian *didgeridoo*, the Sardinian *launeddas* and the Egyptian *arghul*. A few jazz and classical wind and brass players also utilize some form of Circular Breathing. Essentially, Circular Breathing bridges the gap between exhalations. The air stored in the person's cheeks is used as an extra air reserve to play with while they sneak in a breath through their nose. *Bounce Breathing* is an advanced form of Circular Breathing.

CLAVICULAR BREATHING (aka shallow breathing): Clavicle Breathing draws air into the chest area by the raising of the shoulders and collarbone (clavicles). Oxygen reaches only the top third of the lungs; this is the most superficial mode of shallow breathing. *See also Costal Breathing.*

COHERENT BREATHING: Involves breathing at the nominal rate of 5 breaths per minute with equal inhalation and exhalation. This method claims to facilitate circulation and autonomic nervous system balance by creating a wave in the circulatory system, the 'Valsalva Wave' (a term coined by Stephen Elliott).

COSTAL BREATHING (aka *Intercostal Breathing*): A technique in which inspiration and expiration are produced chiefly by movements of the ribs. By expanding the rib cage as the belly comes inward, the breath is forced upward. *Costal* means 'relating to the ribs.'

COUNTING BREATH (BREATHING ISOMETRICS): With the body relaxed, a breathing pattern is maintained. Depth and rhythm may vary. Inhales should last several seconds; exhales are long and slow through your teeth, or with pursed lips, whichever feels comfortable. When in an isometric exercise position, a regular count should be established because holding the breath during exercise is not a good idea—may even be dangerous.

DIAPHRAGMATIC BREATHING: A type of breathing exercise that promotes more effective aeration of the lungs, consisting of moving the diaphragm downward during inhalation and upward with exhalation. *See Belly Breathing.*

HOLOTROPIC BREATHING: Developed by Stanislav Grof as an approach to self-exploration and healing that integrates insights from Eastern spiritual practices as well as modern consciousness research in transpersonal psychology. The method comprises five components: group process, intensified breathing, evocative music, focused bodywork, and expressive drawing.

LATERAL BREATHING: Also called Thoracic Breathing, this technique is the preferred mode during the practice of Pilates. Emphasis is placed on the lateral expansion of the rib cage while maintaining a consistent inward pull of the deep abdominal muscles during both inhalation and exhalation. Lateral Breathing contrasts to Diaphragmatic Breathing.

MERKABA BREATHING: A meditation that consists of 17 breaths; each visualizes a different geometric shape. It is based on the theory that the physical body and spirit can be transported through different dimensions. Also called *Spherical Breathing.*

NADHI SHODHAN PRANAYAMA (aka alternate nostril breathing): Used to de-stress, relax, and concentrate the mind. There are two rounds: with thumb down on the right nostril, one breathes out gently through the left nostril; then inhale through the same nostril. With pinky covering left nostril, breathe out through the right nostril. Inhale through right nostril. Switch. One continues inhaling and exhaling from alternate nostrils.

PATTERNED BREATHING: A learned relaxed and focused breathing technique associated with pregnancy and childbirth. The theory behind breathing patterns is based on the concentration required to focus on the breathing itself, the breath taken in and out of your nose or mouth, or in your nose and out your mouth. The key is to have the breathing feel natural, relaxed, and even at one's own pace.

PERFECT BREATHING: Promotes slower breath and fosters an alert state of mind and a relaxed breathing. The technique is to be used several times a day and should show immediate benefits. Don Campbell, proponent of the method, reports improved mental focus and increased energy. Related practices include: Energy Wave Breathing, Waterfall Breathing, and Imagination Breathing. Also termed "conscious breathing."

PRANAYAMA BREATH: Yogic breathing techniques that help control the "prana" or vital life force (also known as "chi," "qi," or "ki"). The most popular are *Dirga Pranayama* (Three-Part Breath), *Ujjayi Pranayama*, (Ocean Breath), *Nadi Shodhana Pranayama* (Alternate Nostril Breathing), and *Kapalabhati Pranayama* (Light Skull Breathing).

PRANIC BREATHING: A six-step form of breathing that aspires to increase, control, and direct the *prana*, or universal life force. The first step clears negative emotions and limiting beliefs; the second utilizes a highly energizing breathing technique to boost vitality; the third manipulates energy (through scanning, sweeping, and energizing); the fourth step involves energetic hygiene; the fifth step, meditation; the sixth and final step consists of the two very powerful energy-generation exercises.

RECOVERY BREATH: A breathing sequence that Dr. Belisa Vranich teaches to help center oneself before a test or competition, or after an anxiety-producing event in order to calm and recover. It has a vigorous breathing exercise component and a relaxation component. Recovery Breath is also called Active Meditation.

REICHIAN BREATHING (ARMOR): Wilhelm Reich related difficulties in the emotional sphere directly to functional problems on a bodily level as reflected in disturbed breathing; he induced a sense of peace and calm by guiding his patients to focus only on their breath. In Reich's opinion the function of blocking of feeling, motility, and energy in the body creates an *armor* that defends one from threatening internal impulses and from external dangers. In adulthood, this armoring becomes solidified into a person's character structure, a concept that provides one of the cornerstones in the understanding of human functioning.

RESISTANCE BREATHING: The goal is to employ resistance in order to strengthen the muscles used in respiration. Apart from people with breathing disorders, singers, athletes, divers, and martial arts practitioners incorporate resistance breathing into their regimen. Resistance may be provided with the use of respiratory muscle trainers or physical obstacles like pursing the lips to increase resistance during breathing, by suspending the breath.

RHYTHMIC BREATHING: A breathing technique used for running described by Budd Coates in his book *Running on Air*. It centers around the idea that rhythmic breathing increases lung volume; improves awareness and control; helps prevent injury and side stitches; improves running for those with asthma; allows runners to quickly set a pace for quality training and racing; and helps athletes manage muscle cramps.

SITHALI: Referred to as 'tongue hissing' because during the inhale air is drawn in through a protruding tongue folded into a tube. As a result, the air passes over a moist tongue, thereby refreshing the throat. Faster or slower inhalation makes possible variations in loudness and softness and smoothness of a reversed hissing sound. The tongue is drawn back into the mouth and the lips are closed at the end of inhalation. One can breathe out either through the throat or alternately through the nostrils.

SPORTS BREATHING: Breathing techniques related to improved performance during such sports as swimming, biking, or weight lifting, or breathing exercises for endurance and conditioning that train inspiratory and expiratory breathing muscles. Also used after competitive events to reduce stress and tension and induce a calmer state.

TAO YIN BREATHING: Consists of postures, meditation, and breathing patterns to strengthen and relax the back and energize and relax the lumbar area. The goal, explains Taoist Master Mantak Chia, is to achieve harmony between *chi* and external energies and revitalize the body and spirit. Also known as Taoist Yoga.

TAOIST REVERSE BREATHING: Traditionally used by chi kung practitioners, healers, and martial artists, it reverses the natural in-and-out movements of the abdomen present in natural breathing: the abdomen contracts inward during inhalation and relaxes outward during exhalation. When the diaphragm moves downward and the belly contracts inward during inhalation, the resulting pressure in the abdomen "packs" the breath energy; when the diaphragm relaxes upward and the belly relaxes outward during exhalation, the pressure is suddenly released. Reverse Breathing is an advanced technique and should only be undertaken when one is quite comfortable with Abdominal Breathing and with guidance.

THE 4-7-8 BREATHING EXERCISE: An example of a Counting Breath or Breathing Isometric, in this technique one inhales quietly through the nose and exhales audibly through the mouth. The tip of your tongue is placed against the ridge of tissue just behind the upper front teeth through the entire exercise. The inhale is through the nose for 4 counts, breath is held for 7, the exhale is completely through your mouth, making a whoosh sound for 8. The cycle is repeated three more times.

TRANSFORMATIONAL BREATHING: Popularized by Dr. Judith Kravitz, who posits that this technique facilitates the natural healing process for all types of trauma and for beneficial maintenance of optimal health Transformational Breathing is an active exercise that uses the breath to release tension within the body. The breathing technique is a deep breath in through the mouth while inflating the abdomen and a gentle sigh out on the exhale. There is no pause between inhale and exhale.

YOGIC BREATH: Incorporates three types of breathing—

Collarbone (Clavicular) Breathing, Chest Breathing, and Abdominal or Diaphragmatic Breathing—thereby utilizing full-lung capacity. With the inhalation, the abdomen extends forward and the chest is expanded; with the exhalation the chest and the abdomen return to their original position, united into a flowing wave.

BIBLIOGRAPHY AND RECOMMENDED READING

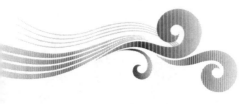

Acharya AU, Joseph K, Kannathal N et al. "Heart Rate Variability," in *Advances in Cardiac Signal Processing.* Springer Verlag, 2007

Altman N. *Oxygen Prescription.* Healing Arts, 2007

Anderson B, Ley R. "Dyspnea during Panic Attacks," *Behavior Modification,* vol. 25, no. 4, pp. 546-54; 2001

Anderson DE, McNeely JD, Windham BG. "Regular slow-breathing exercise effects on blood pressure and breathing patterns at rest," *Journal of Human Hypertension,* vol. 24, no. 12, pp. 807-13; 2010

Beard J. *Thirteen Breaths to Freedom.* Sacred Systems, 2011

Beauchaine T. "Vagal Tone, Development, and Gray's Motivational Theory: Toward an Integrated Model of Autonomic Nervous System Functioning in Psychopathology," *Development and Psychopathology,* vol. 13, no. 2, pp. 183-214; 2001

Bergmark A. "Stability of the lumbar spine. A study in mechanical engineering," *Acta Orthopaedica Scandinavica*, 120 (suppl), pp. 1-54; 1989

Bilchick KC, Berger RD. "Heart rate variability," *Journal of Cardiovascular Electrophysiology*, vol. 17, no. 6, pp. 691-94; 2006

Bohns K, Wiltermuth, SS. "It Hurts When I Do This (or You Do That)," *Journal of Experimental Social Psychology*, vol. 48, pp. 341-45; 2012

Boyle KL, Olinick J, Lewis C. "Clinical Suggestion: The Value of Blowing Up a Balloon," *North American Journal of Sport Physical Therapy*, 5, no. 3, pp. 179-88; 2010

Boyle M. "The Joint-By-Joint Concept (Appendix 1)," in Cook G et al. *Movement: Functional Movement Systems*, 319-21. On-Target Publications, 2012

Brown RP, Gerbarg PL. "Sudarshan Kriya yogic breathing in the treatment of stress, anxiety, and depression: Part I-neurophysiologic model," *Journal of Alternative & Complementary Medicine*, vol. 11, no. 1, pp. 189-201; 2005

Brown RP, Gerbarg PL. *The Healing Power of the Breath: Simple Techniques to Reduce Stress and Anxiety, Enhance Concentration, and Balance Your Emotions.* Shambhala, 2012

Calabrese L. "Volume of Human Lungs" in *The Physics Factbook*, ed. G. Elert, Fair Use Website, 2001

Calais-Germain B. *Anatomy of Breathing.* Eastland Press, 2006

Chiang LC, Ma WF, Huang JL et al. "Effect of relaxation-breathing training on anxiety and asthma signs/symptoms of children with moderate-to-severe asthma: A randomized controlled trial," *International Journal of Nursing Studies*, vol. 46, no. 8, pp. 1061–70; 2009

Conrad A, Müller A, Doberenz S et al. "Psychophysiological Effects of Breathing Instructions for Stress Management," *Applied Psychophysiological Biofeedback*, vol. 32, no. 2, pp. 89–98; 2007

Cook G. *Movement. Functional Movement Systems*. On-Target Publications, 2010

DeSimone ME, Crowe A. "Nonpharmacological approaches in the management of hypertension," *Journal of the American Academy of Nurse Practitioners*, vol. 21, no. 4, pp. 189–96; 2009

Elliot D. *Healing*. Hawk Press, 2010

Farhi D. *The Breathing Book: Good Health and Vitality Through Essential Breath Work*. Holt Paperbacks, 1996

Gallego J, Nsegbe E, Durand, E. "Learning in respiratory control," *Behavior Modification*, vol. 25, no. 4, pp. 495–512; 2001

George R. "Breathe Well and Breathe Often: Defining and Correcting Dysfunctional Breathing Patterns," *Dynamic Chiropractic*, vol. 31, no. 22; 2012

Goldstein DS, Robertson D, Esler M et al. "Dysautonomias: Clinical Disorders of the Autonomic Nervous System," *Annals of Internal Medicine*, vol. 137, no. 9, pp. 753–63; 2002

Grof S, Grof C, Kornfield J. *Holotropic Breathwork*. State University of New York Press, 2010

Guyton AC. *Textbook of Medical Physiology.* W. B. Saunders Company, 1956

Hanh TN. *Breathe, You Are Alive: Sutra on the Full Awareness of Breathing.* Rider & Company, 1992

Hargreave FE, Parameswaran K. "Asthma, COPD and bronchitis are just components of airway disease," *European Respiratory Journal,* vol. 28, no. 2, pp. 264-67; 2006

Hatherley P. *The Internal Development Necessary to Become Loving and Wise.* BalboaPress, 2011

Hendricks G. *Conscious Breathing: Breathwork for Health, Stress Release and Personal Mastery.* Bantam, 2010

Iyengar BKS. *Light on Pranayama: The Yogic Art of Breathing.* Crossroads Publishing, 1985

Jiranjananandanda S. *Prana and Pranayama.* Bihar School of Yoga, 2010

Jones B, Cook G. "Functional Movement System," *Screen II North American Journal of Sports Physical Therapy,* vol. 1 no. 3; 2006

Kapandji IA. "A Forward Head Posture Associated With a 1.44 Greater Rate of Mortality and Chronic Back Pain," in *Physiology of the Joints, III.* Churchill Livingstone, 2008

Kaushik RM, Kaushik R, Mahajan SK et al. "Effects of mental relaxation and slow breathing in essential hypertension," *Complementary therapies in Medicine,* vol. 14, no. 2, pp. 120–26; 2006

Kiesel K, Plisky P, Cook G. "The Selective Functional Movement Assessment: An Integrated Model to Address Regional Interdependence." Course brochure, 2010

Kornfield J, Siegel, D. *Mindfulness and the Brain: A Professional Training in the Science and the Practice of Meditative Awareness.* Sounds True, 2010

Kravitz J. *Breathe Deep Laugh Loudly.* Free Press, 1999

Krieger J. "Respiratory physiology: breathing in normal subjects," in ed. Kryger MH, Roth T, Dement WC. *Principles and practice of sleep medicine.* Saunders W B. Company, 2005

Kubin L, Alheid GF, Zuperku J et al. "Central pathways of pulmonary and lower airway vagal afferents," *Journal of Applied Physiology,* vol. 101, no. 2, p. 618; 2006

La Rovere MT. "Heart rate variability," *Giornale italiano di aritmologia,* vol. 10, no. 1, pp. 20-23; 2007

Lee A, Campbell D. *Perfect Breathing.* Sterling, 2009

Lehrer PM. "Emotionally Triggered Asthma: A Review of Research Literature and Some Hypotheses for Self-Regulation Therapies," *Applied Psychophysiology and Biofeedback,* vol. 23, no. 1, pp. 13-42; 1998

Lewis D. *Free Your Breath, Free Your Life.* Shambhala, 2004

Ley R. "The Modification of Breathing Behavior," *Behavior Modification,* vol. 23, no. 3, pp. 441-79; 1999

Liem KF. "Form and function of lungs: the evolution of air breathing mechanisms," *American Zoologist,* vol. 28, no. 2, p. 739; 1988

Loehr J, Midgow JA. *Breathe in Breathe Out.* Time-Life Books, 1999

Martin D. "Inspiratory muscle strength training improves weaning outcome in failure to wean patients: a randomized trial," *Critical Care,* vol. 15no. 2; 2011

McConnell, Alison. *Breathe Strong, Perform Better.* Human Kinetics, 2011

McGill SM, Sharratt MT, Sequin JP. "Loads on the spinal tissues during simultaneous lifting and ventilator challenge," *Ergonomics,* vol. 38, pp. 1772-92; 1995

Meles E, Giannattasio C, Failla M et al. "Nonpharmacologic treatment of hypertension by respiratory exercise in the home setting 1," *American Journal of Hypertension,* vol. 17, no. 4, pp. 370–74; 2004

Moss MC, Scholey AB. "Oxygen administration enhances memory formation in healthy young adults," *Psychopharmacology,* vol. 124, no. 3, pp. 255–60; 1996

Muench F. *"Breath retraining, the vagus nerve, and depression,"* Perfect Breathing. com

Ohman A, Hamm A, Hugdahl K. "Cognition and the autonomic nervous system: Orienting, anticipation, and conditioning," in *Handbook of psychophysiology.* University Press, 2000

Osho. *Meditation: The First and the Last Freedom.* St. Martin's Griffin, 2004

Parati G, Carretta R. "Device-guided slow breathing as a non-pharmacological approach to antihypertensive treatment: efficacy, problems and perspectives," *American Journal of Hypertension,* vol. 25, no. 1, p. 57; 2007

Perri M. "Rehabilitation of Breathing Patterns, in ed. Liebenson C. *Rehabilitation of the Spine: A Practitioner's Manual.* Lippincott Williams & Wilkins, 2006

Pinna GD, Maestri R, La Rovere MT. "Effect of paced breathing on ventilatory and cardiovascular variability parameters during short-term investigations of autonomic function," *American Journal of Physiology - Heart and Circulatory Physiology*, vol. 290, no. 1, p. H424; 2006

Rama, Ballentine R, Hymes A. *Science of Breathe*. Himalayan Press, 2007

Ray RA. *Your Breathing Body CD*. Sounds True, 2008

Sapolsky R. *Why Zebras Don't Get Ulcers*. Holt Paperbacks, 2004

Saraswati JS. *Prana and Pranayama*. Bihar School of Yoga, 2010

Sarno J. *The Mind-Body Prescription: Healing the Body, Healing the Pain*. Warner, 1999

Scholey AB, Moss MC, Wesnes K. "Oxygen and cognitive performance: the temporal relationship between hyperoxia and enhanced memory," *Psychopharmacology*, vol. 140, no. 1, pp. 123–26; 1998

Schunemann HJ, Dorn J, Grant BJB et al. "Pulmonary Function Is a Long-term Predictor of Mortality in the General Population 29-Year Follow-up of the Buffalo Health Study," *Chest*, vol. 118, no. 3, pp. 656-64; 2000

Seppala EM. "20 Scientific Reasons to Start Meditating Today," *Psychology Today*, 2013

Severinsen SA. *Breatheology*. Idelson Gnocchi, 2010

Smith JC, Abdala APL, Koizumi H et al. "Spatial and functional architecture of the mammalian brain stem respiratory network: a hierarchy of three oscillatory mechanisms," *Journal of Neurophysiology*, vol. 98, no. 6, p. 3370-87; 2007

Taylor K, Orr L, Morningstar J, Ray S. *The Complete*

Breath: A Professional Guide to Health and Wellbeing. Transformations Incorporated, 2012

Telles S, Desiraju T. "Heart rate alternations in different types of pranyamas," *Indian Journal of Physiology and Pharmacology,* vol. 36, no. 4, pp. 287-88; 1993

Telles S, Desiraju T. "Oxygen consumption during pranayamic type of very slow-rate breathing," *Indian Journal of Medical Research,* vol. 94, pp. 357-63; 1991

Van Den Wittenboer G, Van Der Wolf K, Van Dixhoorn J. "Respiratory Variability and Psychological Well-Being in Schoolchildren," *Behavior Modification,* vol. 27, no. 5, pp. 653–70; 2003

Van Dixhoorn J, Duivenvoorden HJ. "Efficacy of Nijmegen questionnaire in recognition of the hyperventilation syndrome," *Journal of Psychosomatic Research,* vol. 29, pp. 199206; 1985

Viskoper R, Shapira I, Priluck R et al. "Nonpharmacologic treatment of resistant hypertensives by Device-Guided slow breathing exercises 1," *American Journal of Hypertension,* vol. 16, no. 6, pp. 484–87; 2003

Weil A. *Breathing: The Master Key to Self-Healing.* Sounds True, 1999

West JB. *Respiratory Physiology: The Essentials.* Lippincott Williams & Wilkins, 2008

Wilhelm FH, Gevirtz R, Roth WT. "Respiratory dysregulation in anxiety, functional cardiac, and pain disorders," *Behavior Modification,* vol. 25, no. 4, pp. 513–45; 2001

Yee, R. *Relaxation and Breathing for Meditation DVD.* Gaiam, 2003.

Establish Your Baseline

1. Vital Lung Capacity:

        Inhale circumference (in inches) <u>34</u>

        Exhale circumference (in inches) <u>30.5</u>

2. Breathhold in Seconds: _____

3. Breaths per Minute: _____

4. Day 1 Resting Heart Rate: _____

5. Stress Level:

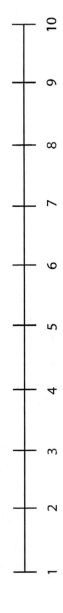

1   2   3   4   5   6   7   8   9   10

LEAST   MOST

6. Pain Level:

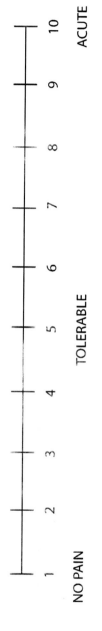

1 2 3 4 5 6 7 8 9 10

NO PAIN   TOLERABLE   ACUTE

7. Energy Level:

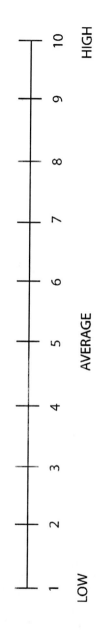

1 2 3 4 5 6 7 8 9 10

LOW   AVERAGE   HIGH

8. Sleep:

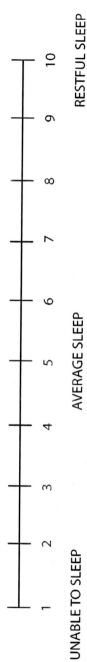

1 2 3 4 5 6 7 8 9 10

UNABLE TO SLEEP   AVERAGE SLEEP   RESTFUL SLEEP

Establish Your Baseline

9.   Mood (Anxiety or Depression):

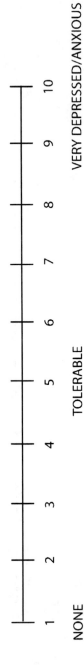

1	2	3	4	5	6	7	8	9	10
NONE				TOLERABLE					VERY DEPRESSED/ANXIOUS

10:   Endurance (self-determined measure):

11:   Cravings:

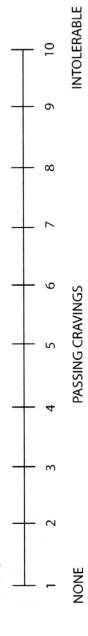

1	2	3	4	5	6	7	8	9	10
NONE				PASSING CRAVINGS					INTOLERABLE

12:   Type of Breather: (check one)

Upper Body Breather (UBB) ☐
Lower Body Breather (LBB) ☐

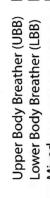

13:   Neck and Shoulder Stiffness/Discomfort:

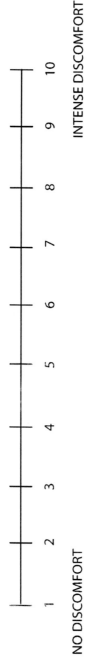

1   2   3   4   5   6   7   8   9   10

NO DISCOMFORT   INTENSE DISCOMFORT

14.   Mental Clarity and Memory:

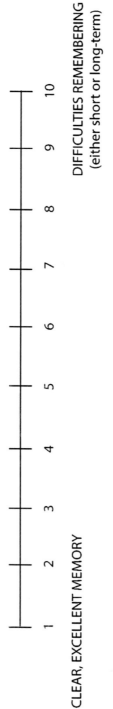

1   2   3   4   5   6   7   8   9   10

CLEAR, EXCELLENT MEMORY   DIFFICULTIES REMEMBERING
                                 (either short or long-term)

15:   Problems with Digestion (constipation, irritable bowel, acid reflux, etc.):

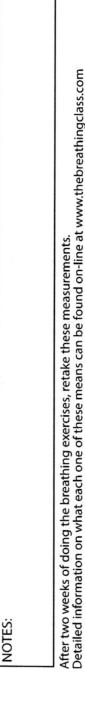

NOTES:

After two weeks of doing the breathing exercises, retake these measurements.
Detailed information on what each one of these means can be found on-line at www.thebreathingclass.com

DAY 1

DAY 2

DAY 3

DAY 4

DAY 5

DAY 6

DAY 7

DAY 8

DAY 9

DAY 10

DAY 11

DAY 12

DAY 13

DAY 14

CPSIA information can be obtained
at www.ICGtesting.com
Printed in the USA
FFOW03n1813230516
24259FF